D1602684

Becoming an Adult Stepchild

Adjusting to a Parent's New Marriage

Becoming an Adult Stepchild

Adjusting to a Parent's New Marriage

Dr. Pearl Ketover Prilik

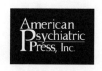

American Psychiatric Press, Inc.

Washington, DC
London, England

American Psychiatric Press, Inc.
1400 K Street, N.W., Washington, DC   20005
www.appi.org

Library of Congress Cataloging-in-Publication Data
Ketover Prilik, Pearl.
    Becoming an adult stepchild : adjusting to a parent's new marriage
    / by Pearl Ketover Prilik. — 1st ed.
        p.   cm.
    Includes index.
    ISBN 0-88048-870-0
    1. Parent and adult child.   2. Adult children—Psychology.
3. Adult children—Family relationships.   4. Remarriage—
Psychological aspects.   5. Stepfamilies—Psychological aspects.
I. Title.
HQ755.86.K47   1998
306.874—dc21   97-24487
                                                                CIP

British Library Cataloguing in Publication Data
A CIP record is available from the British Library.

About the Author

Pearl Ketover Prilik, D.S.W., is the author of *Stepmothering: Another Kind of Love* and *The Art of Stepmothering*. Dr. Prilik brings to her writing varied life and scholarly experience both as a psychotherapist and as a former teacher in areas as diverse as the Virgin Islands and New York City. Dr. Prilik received her undergraduate degree and master's degree in education from New York University. She received her master's and doctoral degree in social welfare from Adelphi University, where she studied the relationship between adolescent exposure to violence and consequent moral reasoning. Dr. Prilik is a candidate in the Postdoctoral Program in Psychoanalysis and Psychotherapy at the Derner Institute for Advanced Psychological Studies in Garden City, New York, where she also has a private practice.

Contents

For D.J.
As always . . .
My constant

Acknowledgments

I acknowledge everyone at American Psychiatric Press who showed how pleasantly and professionally a project can proceed from inception to publication. Special thanks to Claire Reinburg, Editorial Director, the "germinator," provider of the inspiration for this book and its careful nurturer through all stages of growth. Thanks to Alisa Guerzon, Project Editor, for her sharp eyes, precision, and clear "no nonsense" style; to Stacy Jobb, Acquisitions Assistant, for her sunny voice and practical direction; to Pam Harley, Managing Editor, for her accessibility and responsiveness; and to Mark Bloom, Marketing Manager, for his enthusiasm in creating a look and a book from a collection of pages. Special kudos to Anne Friedman, Electronic Pre-Press Manager, for her cover art and design that truly conceptualized in visual form the conflicts, challenges, and joys to be found in this life journey. Thanks to Harvey Klinger, my agent, who handles all the things that most writers don't want to, and probably couldn't, even if they did. Thanks again.

I thank everyone who took time from their own busy lives to read and critique a piece of mine: Margorie Engel, author and President of the Stepfamily Association of America; Jane Marks, author and bride; Dr. Lorelle Saretsky, Director of the Derner Institute's Post-Doctoral Psychotherapy Center; the Vishers, Dr. John and Dr. Emily, founders of the Stepfamily Association of America, for their good wishes.

The reality of human experience brings a richness to a nonfiction text, for it is such experience that both underlies and expands all theoretical understanding. So thanks to all the adult "children" who expanded this field of understanding by sharing their stories, their joys and their sorrows, their frustrations, their questions, and, when they could, their resolutions. Thanks to all the parents of these adults who provided them with a challenge and a remarkable opportunity for continuing intellectual, emotional, and spiritual growth.

Finally, thanks to my son, Joshua, for continuing to glow with that special sunlight that is all his own; to my stepdaughter, Cori, for her unremitting pragmatism; and to my stepson, Brett, who continues to expand his horizons. As always, a final bow to my husband, D.J., who respects a writer's sense of time and in so doing allows the work to continue.

Introduction

If your widowed or divorced parent has recently married or is planning to, you are not alone. Of the 239 million people living in the United States, 80 million—roughly 33%—are involved in stepfamily situations. Within these large numbers are about 20 million "adult stepchildren," of which you are one. Nevertheless, you may already have discovered that somehow you have been overlooked. The bookstore shelves are peppered with volumes about stepparents and stepchildren, but little has been written about adults whose parents decide to get married.

The absence of such help may spring from a vague uneasiness that many adults have in revealing uncomfortable feelings about a parent's marriage. If you do feel uncomfortable, you may wonder why. After all, a little voice may whisper, I am not a child anymore, so why should this be an issue for me? Al, at age 50, said just that:

> My wife just couldn't understand my reaction when my mother said she was going to get married. On the surface, I was happy for her, because I knew she didn't like living alone. The man she was marrying was no stranger to me. They had been friends for years. But all that didn't seem to matter. I couldn't stop thinking about her getting married. It just started preying on my mind all the time, and it wasn't a good feeling. It even affected my marriage for a while; I guess I just withdrew. I didn't want to talk about anything. My wife thought I was kidding at first. "What are you—a baby?" she'd ask me. I didn't need her to make me feel like a fool. I didn't know why my mother's getting married bothered me so much, but it did.

Once I started thinking about adult children, their parents, and marriage, it seemed to me that a parent's marriage did, in fact, raise a host of practical and emotional issues for adult children. But then again, I had written about other aspects of stepfamily life. Could it be, I wondered, that I was a little biased? Was this, in fact, really a topic that concerned many other people? To answer my own question, I began a little "fieldwork," sharing the idea for this book with people in my life.

The reaction was stunning. It seemed that wherever I turned, whoever I told about the book had a story about someone's parent marrying. My internist's wife was struggling with the marriage of her father. My dentist's cousin was shocked by the force of her husband's objections when his widowed mother had married the previous year. The fellow who serviced my car had just had a customer who was complaining about his mother-in-law getting married! A friend with grown children decided to get married, and her daughter wondered about whether to throw her a bridal shower. And so I went ahead, read whatever I could find that had been written about adult children and their relationships with their parents, developed a questionnaire, advertised in local media, and collected responses from the true experts in the field: adults like yourself whose parents had married or were planning to marry.

Finally, here it is—a book devoted to you, the children of a marrying parent. You have discovered that these marriages raise a flurry of things to consider. You may have expected some of these considerations and just need a little help negotiating them, whereas other reactions may have surprised you with the force of an unexpected truck veering around a blind corner.

This book is organized as a resource guide that you may read cover to cover or use to look up particular issues that are of concern to you. Each chapter begins with some questions for you to think about. Throughout each chapter are some practical guidelines for action. The book covers a range of topics from emotional to practical considerations, helping you to untangle what may appear to be a complicated tangle of your parent's actions and your own reactions.

You, Your Parent, and Marriage

★ **Chapter 1** ★

Why Would Your Parent Want to Marry—Now?

Questions to Think About as You Read This Chapter

- As an adult, can you empathize with the problems your parent has faced as a single parent? If you are divorced or widowed yourself, what message does your parent's marriage give to you? Is this a fair and accurate message, or is this message distorted?
- What is your definition of marriage and your understanding of why people marry? Do you apply this definition to your parent's marriage?
- Have you and your parent had similar or different opinions about marriage in the past?
- How did you react to your parent's divorce or the death of your other parent? How did you work through such feelings at the time?

Marriages are like people: somewhat the same across time and society, but at the same time very different at different stages for each individual. Some of the conflicting feelings you may be experiencing concerning your parent's marriage may be rooted in the differences between your and your parent's definition of marriage. If your parent's marriage does not fit into your expectations about why people marry, then you probably will not be able to understand and support your parent's decision; this was a difficulty Pat faced:

> It was difficult for Pat to accept that her mother had "chosen another man" after the death of Pat's father. Instead, Pat interpreted her mother's decision to marry as something that had been forced on her. She preferred to believe that her mother went through with the marriage simply because she had already promised to do so and could not bring herself to decide otherwise, no matter how much she might have wanted to. Pat would like to hear her mother validate her understanding of the reasons for the marriage and say, "I only married him because he was waiting for me."

One way to work toward identifying with your parent's decision to marry is to try to understand what life has been like for him or her since becoming single again. The loss of a spouse through either death or divorce is widely acknowledged as an extraordinarily stressful life event. A parent suddenly loses his or her identity as one member of a married couple, sometimes after decades of having thought of himself or herself in that way. After the end of their marriage, widowed or divorced parents may feel adrift and unsure of who they are. Different dynamics are at play in the situations widowed or divorced parents face.

Life as a Single Parent

Long-Married Parents Who Divorce

The effect of divorce on older parents may be far more devastating than it is on younger parents, and their suffering will affect their children and their relationship with them.

Feeling of failure. When divorce occurs during a parent's middle years or beyond, it may be perceived as a failure or a waste of years, prompting feelings of sadness and even depression in the parent. This drastic change comes at a time when the parent is just beginning to take stock of his or her worth and review and evaluate his or her life's achievements.

Economic hardship. The economic hardships of divorce are no easier to cope with for long-married couples than for those married a shorter time. Unless assets have been set aside, parents from midlife on may feel a terrible anxiety that they will not be able to make it alone.

Lack of peer support. The long-married parent typically faces a lack of social support from friends who may be less accepting of divorce. His or her peers may have been taught that staying in an unhappy marriage is more acceptable than breaking up a family through divorce. The parent may even face hostility from peers who are grieving the death of a spouse and cannot understand why a couple would voluntarily dissolve their marriage.

Long-Married Parents Whose Spouses Die

Long-married parents grieving the death of a spouse face problems similar to those of divorced parents but with a different twist. Initial adjustment to their single life may be easier in that they are more likely to receive both emotional and practical support from their family and friends and financial support from life insurance settlements. However, long-term challenges may pose more of a difficulty.

Idealizing marriage or deceased spouse. Unlike divorced parents who may think of their marriage as having been a failure, newly widowed parents may idealize both their marriage and their departed spouse. Such idealization may keep them from moving forward into a new lifestyle or relationship, because any changes they make or new potential mates they meet will be measured against the original relationship or mate and will be perceived as not making the grade.

Difficulty managing funds. Although widowed parents may experience less economic hardship than do divorced parents, especially at first with life insurance and pension settlements, they may have difficulty unilaterally making financial decisions after a lifetime of either consulting with their spouse on financial matters or, in some cases, leaving financial matters completely to their spouse.

Lack of support from married friends. Although grieving parents do not encounter the stigma of being divorced, nor experience their peers as finding fault with their perceived inability to make a marriage work, they encounter other hurtful—and surprising—difficulties as they seek social support from their married friends. Because many people are uncomfortable with grief, widows and widowers may find themselves not included in their friend's activities.

Physical challenges.   Older, newly widowed parents may find it difficult to adapt to an independent lifestyle because they are not as physically able as when they were younger. They may have less physical mobility, be more restricted in when and how far they can drive (for example, they may not be able to drive at night), and be limited in the new activities they can pursue through which they can seek companionship.

Short-Married or Never-Married Parents

Parents who were married for only a short time may still be seeking the security of commitment and may fear being abandoned again. On the other hand, parents who were never married may continue to harbor the lost dream of a unified family. Parents who had short-term marriages or who never married may have high expectations when they marry later in life and about the role their adult children will play in their marriage.

For children who do not remember their parent as part of a couple, marriage may either feed or clash with their own buried fantasies of "family." Some adults, like their parents, may still long for the fantasy of the unified original family and find themselves disturbingly hostile to their parent's marriage. Other adults may find that the notion of a married parent is simply alien to their way of thinking and feel that in some way their own sense of identity is shaken.

What Your Parent May Be Looking for in Marriage

As noted above, people marry at different times for different reasons. Young couples typically marry with the intention of growing older together and building a life—including raising children—together. More mature couples at the peak of their professional careers may marry to have someone with whom to share leisure time and to combat the stress of their respective work endeavors. Older couples may marry for companionship, to avoid the difficulties of single life and potential loneliness, and to have a compatriot who can understand the depths of loss as well as the joyful highs one experiences in a lifetime. Thus, a parent who once vowed never to marry again might change his or her view at a different stage of life, much to the shock of his or her now grown children. This was the case with Eliot, as he relates in the following story:

> My mother always swore she would never get married again. In fact, when I was in junior high school, I remember that my mother's friends used to kid around and say that my mother's name was "Mrs. I'm Not Getting Married Again." She did make a lot of what then seemed to be good-natured jokes about marriage—things like, "I tried it once and it didn't agree with me," or things that embarrassed me in front of my friends like, "The only good thing to come out of my marriage was Eliot." Anyway, I guess as time went along, I sort of believed that what she was saying was the way that she felt. She didn't even go out on dates or anything.
>
> So when she called me up and told me she had something to talk to me about, I thought she was sick or something. Anyway, when we got together and she introduced me to this guy and told me she was getting married, I didn't even get it at first. I was just sitting there not saying anything. All I can say is that it was a complete shock. I'm not sure how I feel; it's like asking me how I'd feel about my mother flying around the state: I don't have much of a feeling; it's still such a bizarre idea.

Ken, a young man in his mid-20s, expressed a similar reaction to his mother's impending marriage:

> I didn't have any real memories of my mother ever being married. I mean, I knew she had been divorced when I was 5, but this didn't have any personal meaning for me. It had been just Mom for my entire life: Mom as a separate and distinct person from everyone else. I don't suppose I gave it much thought at all until she told me that she was thinking about getting married. The only way I can put it is that marriage and Mom just didn't go together. It just felt completely off.

A parent may wait until his or her children are settled before even beginning to socialize. This seemed to be the case with Eliot's mother, who waited until Eliot had graduated from professional school and had begun his career before she began to date. If your circumstances are similar to Eliot's, consider that people—including your parent—change over time. Marriage for an independent woman with grown children has decidedly different aspects than marriage for a young single mother!

★ Remember that marriage may be better for your parent's health. Studies have shown that married couples live longer, happier, and ultimately healthier lives than adults living alone.

★ Accept that your parent is a separate individual from you; your ability to accept your parent's choices—especially of a lifetime partner—is a major accomplishment in your personal growth.

★ Do not compare yourself and your parent in terms of mutual definitions of marriage. Your parent is at a different life stage and is a separate and unique individual with his or her own background of life experience. Viewed from this perspective of personal differences, you and your parent likely will have different definitions of marriage that are appropriate to stage of life and personal preferences.

★ Do some reading, watch a film, or rent some videos, and think about the reasons that people marry at different times of their lives.

Is It Appropriate for You to Approve or Disapprove of Your Parent's Marriage?

You may perceive that your parent is explicitly—or implicitly—asking you, his or her child, to approve or disapprove of the marriage. The concept of your judging your parent's action may engender the feeling in you that everything that appears normal is now being stood on its ear. The way out of this dilemma is to remember that you are there to witness this event, not to sanctify it or give your permission for it; you are being asked to do nothing more than share in the day. Any wedding is an occasion for others—including children of one of the participants—to acknowledge publicly an already-established relationship.

Another aspect to being (even implicitly) asked your opinion of your parent's wedding is that this may signal the first time you as an adult child and your parent publicly acknowledge each other as adults whose lives are both united and autonomous.

When your parent asks for your approval, it may indicate a turn-around in the parent-child relationship that may have occurred long ago when you lived alone with your parent and took on some of the responsibilities of your missing parent. A parent's marriage may be an ideal, although difficult, opportunity for you as an adult child to step out of the role of being solely responsible for your parent's emotional well-being. Actually, stepping away from accepting the role of judge in your parent's life may bring new insights to you. You may realize as an adult child that you and your parent are capable of having loving relationships that operate to enhance rather than threaten both your and your parent's relationships.

Wedding Ceremonies as Rituals

Before looking at your perspective on marriage, which has evolved from your personal experiences, let's explore what weddings, in general, are all about. Like all other ceremonies, weddings are events that have been ritu-alized by society. To begin to understand your parent's wedding, it is es-sential to understand the role such rituals play. Rituals are a society's way of formally recognizing a change in a component of its social structure—in this case, the family—and simultaneously making that change known to other members of that society. Family rituals are especially powerful. They are the way that a family proclaims, "This is who we are!" A wedding, then, could be seen as the very first family ritual. "But," you might ask, "how can my parent's upcoming wedding be a first ritual in a family that has already existed?" Further, digging a little deeper into this dilemma, if this wedding is indeed this new couple's first family ritual, where does that leave you, the child of your parent's first family?

Before answering that question, let's examine the purpose of the wedding ceremony itself to highlight what, if anything, is troubling to you about it. A wedding proclaims that

1. Two people now form a couple.
2. The partners make certain promises to each other.
3. The couple has a binding, loving relationship that is now socially and legally recognized.

Because any one of these proclamations may kick up some trouble for you as the adult child, let's examine them one at a time.

Two People Now Form a Couple

The idea of your parent as part of a new couple may be unsettling to you as your parent's child, especially because this new couple is not the original parental couple. Before hearing about their impending marriage, when your parent and his or her intended spouse were dating, you probably did not find your parent's being part of a new couple threatening. You may have viewed your parent's dating simply as something that a solitary parent did for enjoyment, rather like a hobby. However, once their marriage was announced, you saw this couple in a new light.

The way in which you ultimately come to view the new couple will evolve and may take a variety of forms. You may come to view the couple as simply an extension of the dating situation—your parent and a person with whom he or she enjoys companionship. You may come to think about the couple as older friends with whom you share a special and unique bond. You may come to think about your parent and his or her spouse as an extended family unit connected to the family by your relationship with your parent. You may even come to view the new couple as parents or as a grandparenting couple.

> Shortly after Jane's mother passed away, her elderly father married Anna. Jane greeted the marriage with mixed feelings. On the one hand, Jane was pleased that her father seemed happy after a painful time, and, on the other hand, Jane was vaguely discomfited by the quickness of the marriage. Jane's three children were also a bit confused about their relationship to this new woman. Anna swept into their lives and seemed delighted with the prospect of being able to be a grandmother because she had no children of her own. Within 2 years of the marriage, Jane's father passed away, and Anna continued to be a grandmother to the children. Anna helped Jane through the death of her father and became the only grandparent to Jane's children because her husband's parents were both deceased.

The Partners Make Certain Promises to Each Other

The promises that members of a couple make to each other in your presence may take on either a bittersweet or simply a bitter cast. If you have not resolved lingering resentments about your sense of betrayal by the parent who is now marrying, these promises may echo hollowly. On the other hand, you should realize some elemental facts about your parents: 1) they were a couple before they were your family, 2) they were individuals before they were a couple, and, perhaps most important, 3) your parent is a unique individual rather than a creation of your own wishes and desires. Understanding that your parent is a unique individual as well as your parent may help you clarify and enhance your own sense of being an individual as well as a member of a family. You will then be able to share in your parent's happy occasion without feeling that there is a demand on you to give anything more than your very sincere good wishes. Working through the task of separating from your parent involves coming to a point where you can not only be your own person but also allow your parent to be his or her own person rather than the someone you may need him or her to be (see Chapter 2).

The Couple Has a Socially and Legally Recognized Relationship

A parent's marriage is a statement of commitment to another person. Your parent now proclaims his or her devotion to a person in a way that is socially and legally recognized by the community. The idea of your parent marrying another person may raise a host of issues for you as an adult child. If you have unresolved and perhaps long-buried childhood fantasies of reconciliation (between your parents), this marriage may seem to be a not-too-veiled insult. If the notion of your parent's union as socially and legally sanctioned is unsettling for you, you may have to think about what is actually troubling you. Perhaps you have shelved your thinking about your parent's relationship with the person he or she is marrying and now find that you are hit with a barrage of stored emotions. It is also not uncommon for an adult child to have questions about inheritances and family possessions, which are disturbing to think about. While your parent was unmarried, there may have been no need to discuss dispersion of assets and favorite family possessions. However, a parent's marriage may raise questions and thus seem to pressure an adult child to think about a parent's demise. Furthermore, what may have seemed understood and natural when a parent was unmarried may now be uncertain. Most uncomfortable may be the feeling that such discussions simply cannot be brought up, and a disturbing anxiety begins to hover over your relationship with your parent.

A parent's marriage forces an adult child to examine his or her sense of entitlement; questions arise about what belongs to a parent and what belongs to you as the child of that parent. You may have never had the opportunity to think about these questions. Some adults feel that the parents' possessions belong to the children as part of a large family pot, other adults feel that the parents' possessions are for the parents to do with as they wish, and still other adults fall somewhere in the middle. Whether you have a clear idea of where you fall on this spectrum or whether you have never thought of such issues, a parent's marriage can be thought of as an opportunity for some advanced thinking.

You and Your Parent's Marriage

So where does all this leave you and your thoughts on marriage? Your idea of what constitutes a marriage and why people marry is largely based on what you witnessed within your own family—while your parents were married, how they were separated (whether through death, divorce, or abandonment), and what happened once they were separated. If your parents were divorced, then your perspective will differ from that of an individual who had one parent die. These experiences will then form your reaction to subsequent marriages: your siblings', your parent's second (or more) marriage, and even your own marriage.

Different Reactions Among Siblings

Even though you and your siblings shared similar family experiences, your reactions to your parent's marriage can be completely different. Claire, a 57-year-old attorney, thought she would be thrilled when her father decided to marry, but she had quite a different reaction when her father actually made his announcement. She also received a second surprise when she compared her reaction with that of her sister:

> My father had been dating a lovely and, I might add, much younger woman. Dad was almost 80, and my sister and I had a good time privately chuckling over what we called his "antics." Then, one night when we were all out eating dinner, he announced his engagement. My sister was hugging and kissing him and his bride-to-be, but I was simply para-

lyzed; I couldn't move. Of course, I did force myself to try to say something appropriate, but I was so overcome by this enormous rage that I had to leave the table. A short time later, I made some sort of excuse and went home before dessert was served.

Claire was doubly surprised by her father's announcement. First, she was surprised at the intensity of her negative feelings about the marriage, and second, she was surprised by her sister's acceptance:

If you had asked me before all this happened who would have had the harder time adjusting, I would have said my sister without a moment's hesitation. My sister had always been Daddy's little girl. Who would have ever thought it would be my sister hugging and toasting everyone and me hightailing out to my car?

Sometimes a parent's marriage enlivens old and unresolved wishes and desires. In Claire's case, although she ostensibly had accepted that her "sister had always been Daddy's little girl," Claire may have harbored a long-held fantasy that someday her turn would come. For Claire, her father's marriage may have triggered a sense of deprivation that forced her to deal with her perhaps repressed feelings of abandonment by her father, who had from this perspective "left her" for her mother, her sister, and now another and nonrelated female! Whereas Claire might have been able to contain her "negative feelings," as she puts them, for her mother and sister, this long-simmering rage unexpectedly bubbled to the surface with her father's announcement of marriage.

Do not be surprised if your siblings or, for that matter, other family members react very differently from yourself to the news of your parent's marriage. Your reaction will be ultimately an expression of the strengths, weaknesses, fears, and hopes that are a part of your relationship with your parent and as such will be different from that of anyone else.

★ Try not to "prove your point" to your siblings about your feelings about the marriage. Obviously in your lives together you have had other occasions where you have not seen a situation in the same way. Use this as an opportunity to explore your unique perspective and to understand yourself and yourself in relation to others better.

Children Whose Parents Have Divorced

Children of divorced parents bring conflicting emotions to their view of marriage. One emotion is the fear of abandonment. If children were young when their parents divorced, it would not have been unusual for them to feel their parent left them as well. This reaction can lead to a real sense of abandonment, which must be dealt with by both parents.

Second, children of divorced parents can have many ambivalent feelings toward each parent, feelings that resurface when one or another parent decides to marry. A child, even a young child, may strongly identify with the pain of the "left" parent. That sense of identification can become even stronger when that child becomes an adult; for example, a happily married woman may so identify with her abandoned mother that she becomes anxious by fearing her own abandonment, even though she has no real grounds for such fears. An adult child may find that feelings of bitterness, anger, rage, anxiety, and depression are triggered when the abandoning parent marries. Such unpleasant feelings may be a condensed mixture of feelings that the adult child has internalized from the aggrieved parent, taken on as his or her own, and added to his or her own personal grievances against the parent viewed as abandoning.

Third, a child of divorced parents is buffeted by loyalty issues throughout childhood and into adulthood. Even if a child sees both parents regularly under the most optimum, amicable conditions, that child still loses the opportunity to live in a family that lives, grows, and shares a family history under one roof. Conditions following a divorce are never ideal, and in such situations, children of all ages have to confront loyalty issues as they live with the parent who has custody and visit the other.

The loyalty issues of children of divorced parents are difficult. These children often feel that positive feelings for one parent are in conflict with the other parent's perspective. Such conflicts are especially difficult for children who are in the process of their own emotional development, formulating their identity based in part on aspects of their parents' personalities and their feelings for them. Over time, a child will most likely find a way to cope with these conflicts that is more or less satisfying to the parents and to the child's own view of self. Children in this situation may deny feelings, may act out their feelings, or may learn to negotiate the conflict between the individual parents and themselves. Nevertheless, when children feel that having affectionate feelings for one parent betrays the other parent, the ongoing tension may flare when a parent decides to marry. An adult child may decide to perpetuate the accommodations he or she has learned to make throughout his or her relationships with the parents and become more entrenched in defending a parent who he or she perceives as aggrieved. On the other hand, an adult child may realize that, for too long, his or her feelings for a parent have been constrained by a sense of loyalty that was inappropriate and is now outdated. The adult child may find that his or her parent's marriage provides an opportunity to either switch allegiances or confront a parent who has demanded "loyalty" and attempt to finally end the conflict.

> David's parents divorced when he was a young child. As a child, David heard many negative things about his father from his mother's family, but he never blamed his father for the consequences that David, his mother, and his siblings seemed to suffer after the divorce. David pushed aside criticisms of his father and his father's lack of financial or emotional support and enjoyed his occasional visits with him. When David's father recently married for the third time, David found himself recognizing the hurt that he felt. The father's third marriage suddenly made his father seem to have more than his share, whereas David was left with so very little. David had kept his father safe from his own blame since his parents' divorce, but with his father's marriage, David found that he very much wanted his father to accept responsibility for having made David's life very difficult in order to enjoy his own pleasures.

Fourth, children of divorced parents tend to develop skepticism about the viability of marriage as well as general anxiety about relationships and trusting others. These biases are then tapped into as they react to their parents' impending marriages. Three different issues are included in the adult child's skepticism. First, the adult child may question the parent's ability to stay married. The parent has been viewed as part of a separated couple rather than as part of a functioning unit. Second, the adult child may wonder whether the parent has the perseverance to make any marriage work. An adult child may never have fully understood the reasons for the failure of the parent's marriage. If the parent never married, then such questions about the parent's capability to form a stable marriage may be exacerbated. Finally, the adult child may question the viability of marriage as an institution. With little or no personal experience of a working couple and the positive attributes that marriage may offer, an adult child may have a distorted impression of marriage as an institution. Simply put, if he or she could not trust his or her own parents to stay together and make a go of it, he or she may wonder how his or her parent will be able to carry off this new marriage.

> Dinah's parents divorced when Dinah was 2 years old. They had been separated for about a year before their divorce. After their divorce, Dinah did not see her father until she was 19. In the years between, Dinah and her mother lived a "single girls' life" together. Dinah often boasted to her friends that her mother was more of a friend than a mother and that they did just fine without anyone's help. Through the years, Dinah's mother would joke about marriage, calling it "a man's invention." The clear implication to Dinah was that they could do just fine without any "outside" help. When Dinah was 23, she returned from graduate school to learn of her mother's announcement of marriage. Dinah found it difficult to accept the idea of her mother's marriage. She had grown up with an underlying theme of distrust of men and of marriage as an outmoded institution designed to constrain women's independence.

In some cases, adult children whose parents have been divorced can easily accept a parent's marriage because they saw the unhappiness their parent lived with for years. It is enough for them that their parent seems happy:

> Hank, age 29 years, was aware that his father had had a difficult marriage with his mother, who was an alcoholic; yet, Hank's father "hung in there" despite the fact that his mother refused to seek help, that other marital problems were exacerbated by her addiction, and that his own analysis finally confirmed that their differences were irreconcilable. Despite these extreme difficulties, Hank's father waited until all the children were self-sufficient adults before getting a divorce. Shortly after Hank's parents were divorced, Hank's father met and married a young woman, not much older than his children. However, Hank had no problem with the marriage because it felt good to see his father happy. The couple was married in Las Vegas, with Hank and his two brothers in attendance.

Children Whose Parent Has Died

Children who have had one parent die also have several issues with which to deal. One is the degree of responsibility they feel for their surviving parent, which can vary according to the parent's level of independence and the other factors operating in the child's life. If you were a child when your parent died, you may have felt either compelled to try to take care of your surviving parent—which left you feeling overburdened—or frightened and unprotected. If you were an adult at the time, your sense of responsibility toward your surviving parent may have been even stronger, leading you at times to feel the pull of guilt or resentment as your parent's needs inevitably clashed with your own responsibilities and desires.

Second, you may find that you have not fully resolved your feelings of grief from losing your surviving parent and that these feelings surge within you when your parent decides to marry. At the time of your parent's death, you may have felt that you were left to cope alone without the social structure and support offered to your grieving parent. Typically, at the time of the death, your surviving parent received more attention as the grieving widow or widower than you did as the child; this was probably based on family's and friend's misunderstandings about the needs of children and their own grieving process. For example, some children have reported being told to "go outside and play" shortly after the death of their parent. Isolated from other grieving relatives, children often felt alone with their grief and had to sort out their complicated feelings on their own or with age-mates who were ill-equipped to respond.

When the surviving parent decides to marry, the adult child may feel once again left to cope alone with the loss of both parents. The adult child may feel a responsibility to carry on the memory of the deceased parent, and the living parent may be viewed as "lost" to the new spouse.

In addition to these feelings of grief for the departed parent, the death of a parent may harshly affect a child's perspective about marriage. In a very real and compelling way, a child may come to view marriage and the bonds between family members as fragile and/or unpredictable. The grief felt by a child that he or she continues to bear may come from longing for the view of stability that existed before the parent's death. Marriage may seem to be a threatening proposition with a sizable dose of anxiety that leads to a keenly felt sense of inevitable loss.

Although you always remain a child of your parents, regardless of your age, it is important to rethink your parent's death from an adult perspective and understand that no one "gets over" anyone in the sense of obliterating that person from his or her life. People do move on in life; experiences that once had a significant impact assume a different level of importance as time goes on. Losses cannot remain raw, and grieving cannot, and should not, go on forever. If you can, let your parent's marriage be an opportunity for you to move forward from grieving for the loss of your parent. Emily, in the following example, had reached that point:

> Emily, who just turned age 50, described her mother's wedding in loving and glowing terms. "It was a small family affair. They had both met at church many, many years ago when both their spouses were still living, and so being married there felt appropriate to them. My mother bought the most expensive dress that she's ever owned."
>
> The wedding felt appropriate for Emily as well. Seeing her mother being married in the familiar church that Emily's father had attended was comforting and "right" for Emily. She understood her mother's special efforts (for example, buying an expensive dress) as an expression of her mother's happiness and good feelings about herself.

It is always a relief to see a parent whom we truly love feeling happy and good about himself or herself. For Emily, it was as though her mother's new union was sanctioned by the couple's departed spouses because they had known each other previously. A parent's wedding can be easier to accept when the deceased parents had known and liked each other. It may be that these circumstances relieve some unconscious responsibility and loyalty conflicts an adult child feels and allows him or her to react positively to this chance of his or her parent's being happy.

In the case of either divorce or death, try to see your parent's new marriage as a testament of hope. In the case of marriage interrupted by death, the new marriage can be a nod of recognition to your deceased parent and his or her part in your parent's positive view of marriage itself. As adults, we can understand that a parent's choosing a new spouse is not an attempt to replace the original spouse, but rather a choice based on the attraction another individual holds for him or her. In cases of marriage ended by divorce, the "nod" may be that, whatever damage was done, no matter how grievous, it was not irreparable. If your parent was in a particularly bad marriage and swore never to marry again, you may view your parent's decision to marry as an action signifying that he or she no longer blames your other parent for wrongs done.

★ Create some type of ritual to memorialize your original parents' marriage. Envision yourself pressing their marriage under glass, like a beautiful flower to be preserved forever. You are not letting it go; you are remembering the past and sharing the present.

★ Take your parent's marriage as an opportunity to release feelings about your parent's death or divorce that may have held you in their grip.

Chapter 2

Making Sense of the Complex Web of Childhood Emotions

Questions to Think About as You Read This Chapter

- What kind of relationship have you had with your parent during the past several years? Has this relationship been more or less the same throughout your life?
- Is your relationship with your parent satisfactory? Are you concerned that this relationship will in some way change?
- Is your relationship with your parent unsatisfactory? Are you concerned that this relationship will in some way worsen?
- What was your relationship with your other parent? How are your feelings for your other parent, whether deceased or divorced, affecting your feelings about this marriage?
- What do you, as an adult, think about how adult parent and adult child relationships should be? What can you do, as an adult, to help bring about such a relationship between yourself and your parent?

As an adult child, you have already had to make major adaptations in your relationship with your parent or parents in your family of origin following their initial separation. When parents divorce or one parent dies, the child's relationship with both parents or the surviving parent undergoes a major transition. Then, when a parent decides to marry, the adult child faces yet another major transition; the difficulty in making that transition can be that some unwelcome baggage from the past remains.

Why Do I Feel So Angry?

A common reaction to a parent's announcement of marriage is fierce, often inexplicable anger. The probable source of this anger—the child's feelings of abandonment, whether by the parent who died or left or by the parent the child never knew—is well hidden. Instead, those feelings of abandonment masquerade in the adult behind a mask of anger toward the marrying parent and/or the new spouse for what is perceived as a new betrayal of the other parent. However, that sense of betrayal is more accurately centered within the adult child; it is the child who felt betrayed by the dissolution of the parents' union and who felt deprived of a family by divorce, death, or abandonment. That child's anger, born in the past, now finds its voice in the adult as the parent finds a new partner. It is as though the dissolution of the child's family is once again brought into the spotlight and reenacted with the parent's decision to marry. Now, in a compelling and real way, any deeply buried fantasies of reconciliation may rise to the surface with all the old longing. The new marriage is now the target of this deeply felt disappointment that things truly never will be the way they were or the way the adult child wishes they could be.

Unresolved feelings of anger and abandonment can cause adult children to act out in a way they know will hurt their parent, for this remains the only way they can express pain they feel inside, as in the following three examples. In most cases, the expression of that anger is not in anyone's best interests.

> Ted's father had abruptly left his mother and moved to another country when Ted was in his 20s. The move left Ted's mother financially and emotionally devastated. When the father married several years later, Ted rallied his six siblings to boycott the wedding.

> Lily was upset when her mother decided to marry shortly after Lily's father died but was unable to voice her concerns. Instead, she acted out

her feelings by refusing to allow her 8-year-old daughter to attend the ceremony. She told her mother, "It just isn't possible; after all, she has her monthly piano recital on that very same day." Later, Lily was able to admit that she was still very angry at how quickly her mother had decided to remarry after her father's death.

Cindy was furious when her mother decided to get married. Although she was angry, she accepted her mother's invitation to be in the bridal party and expected that she would "be able to make the best of it." At the wedding, Cindy became drunk and found that she "just hated the whole wedding from beginning to end."

★ If you feel angry, bitter, or rageful at your parent, try to focus on the source of those feelings. Don't leave things simply at "I'm angry because my mother hurt Dad" or "Mom's been a wreck since my father left." Search for what you feel was wrong about the actions of the parent who has disappointed you, because at the root of your bitterness or anger you will find your own disappointment lurking.

The Child in You Steps Forward

Just when you as an adult have more or less completed separating from your parents and becoming an individual in your own right, your parent marries. The marriage forms a new family. This new family business may cause you to reexamine your relationship with your parent, and with this reexamination comes a resurgence of childhood anxieties, wishes, and fears. In a very real sense, the marriage of a parent encourages an adult child to think about how he or she fits into this new family grouping as the child of the marrying parent, which can be very unsettling. This dynamic is combined with the unsettling practical and psychological realities of integrating someone new into the parental role—whether in the literal or figurative sense.

The Process of Separating From Your Parent

Through all the conflicting feelings that you may have felt or are feeling right now about your parent's marriage, you may wonder why you are taking all this quite so personally. But think about it—it would be difficult for you not to take your parent's marriage personally. After all, your relationship with your parent was your first relationship with another person and as such set the stage for all your relationships that followed. How well you have moved from a relationship characterized by total dependency on your parent to one in which you are both individuals relating interdependently will be a major factor in how you cope with your parent's marriage. To understand the dynamics of this maturation process, let's take a closer look at how the nature of your relationship with your parent changes over time.

Your relationship with your parents began as one of total dependence. You probably did not know where you left off and they began. Whoever parented you had to meet your most basic needs of food, warmth, and so forth to guarantee your survival. However, regardless of how attuned your parents may or may not have been to you, no infant can be perfectly cared for. A gap between the baby's needs and the parents' ability to fulfill those needs is inevitable. Thus, at times, you, like all babies, experienced a state of bliss in which your needs may have appeared to be fulfilled only by thinking about them, but at other times, you experienced disappointment, anger, and fear during that gap between your need and its fulfillment. You experienced all these feelings—from bliss and contentment to rage and frustration. Over time, you became better able to soothe yourself and, little by little, to meet some of your own needs. You began to feed yourself, to walk, to talk, and to grow increasingly less dependent on those who parented you for survival. As these physical markers of self-sufficiency increased, psychological developments occurred simultaneously.

As you matured into adulthood, one of the hallmarks of that maturity was the ability to be aware that the provocative wish to merge with another person harks back to those early days of infancy. As a mature adult, you realize that perfect harmony between two individuals has a magical quality that is a residue of those earliest days. You also realize that relationships between individuals are marked by attunements and misattunements bridged by an ability to communicate.

One of the struggles faced by many adults is the ability to separate from parents without feeling cut off and the ability to relate to parents without feeling overwhelmed or engulfed by them. In a very real way, negotiating a pathway between being alone and being swallowed up is a central task in reaching adulthood. So, what does all this have to do with your parent marrying?

How well you fared in completing the task of separating from the image of fantasy parents who you created and internalized as part of your personality and who have the magical ability to satisfy your every need will play a major role in how you cope with your parent's marriage.

If you are feeling emotional about your parent's marriage for reasons you cannot quite put your finger on, chances are that some of your old inner others have sprung up and are clamoring for your attention. For example, you may be feeling fear, that is, being afraid that your parent may abandon you in favor of this new person. You may be reacting with hostility or anger, even rage, because you sense that you and your needs are being displaced by the needs of a new loved one in your parent's life. You may be feeling that you have not received "enough" of some undefined quality from your parent and that now you may never have a chance to redress this deficit. Alternatively, you may be feeling deprived, lonely, sad, depressed, disappointed, or on edge because you sense that something was, is, or will be in danger of being lost.

Because a parent's marriage may cause old insecurities residing either slightly or deeply beneath the surface to rise, it is useful to use the occasion of your parent's marriage as an opportunity for self-exploration. Think about other times in your life that you have let go and experienced growth. If you have not experienced letting go and growing, think about familiar situations such as a baby's need to let go of a parent's hand in order to move away. We smile as we watch a toddler struggle with the conflicting desire between wanting to move away from a parent and being terrified of his or her own untested ability; we smile because we know he or she is capable. We know that the parent won't disappear if the child moves away. Try to recapture your sense of having a choice—the choice to return to dependency and the way things have always been or to move forward. The feelings that your parent's marriage inspires may open new doors for relating to your parents, to others, and to yourself, in ways that you, like that toddler, have never imagined before and yet are truly capable of experiencing.

★ Think about the changes in your relationship with your parent through the years. Record these changes in some way so that you can actually look at them. Make a timeline or chart, or simply list them.

Reexperiencing an Infantile Sense of Helplessness

Another source of your discomfort as you try to adjust to your parent's marriage could be your sense of lack of control over the entrance of this new individual into your life in an intimate role—whether the intimacy is limited to your parent or affects you directly. To understand your feelings more clearly, think about the beginning of your life as an infant, when you lived in a blur of sensations and were unaware of where you ended and others began. If you are feeling a bit helpless about your parent's decision to marry, it may help to remember that although as an infant you were totally dependent on others for your physical and psychological well-being, you are now at the other end of the spectrum—a mature adult capable of meeting a wide range of your own needs. Your parent's choice of a new partner and his or her impending marriage to that person may threaten to pull you back from that secure end of the adult spectrum toward the direction of that long-ago helpless infant. However, your relationships with others are no longer determined by forces outside your control or understanding, as they were so very long ago. If you recognize the feeling as a throwback to the distant past rather than a present-day reality, you may have found a way to feel much more comfortable.

Fearing the Loss of Your Parent as a Constant in Your Life

As an adult, you have more than likely been focusing on your own life: building a career, forming relationships, perhaps even building a family of your own. Yet somewhere your parent has always been "out there" as a building block in the foundation of your life. Then, when your parent announces his or her intention to marry—or even more startlingly, breaks the news of a marriage that has already taken place—your sense of constancy founded in your parent is shaken. To understand how to cope with this sudden sense of shifting sands, you must first understand why having that sense of constancy is so important.

One of the interesting quirks about ourselves as human beings is that although we can count on relatively few things to remain the same, we nonetheless enjoy consistency. In fact, we strive to maintain our sense of personal security by believing that we can predict what will come next. One task in maturing into an adult, however, is realizing that life is simply not as predictable as we might like—or might think we would like—it to be.

The sense of security in a parent-child relationship is twofold and is based on myriad interactions: 1) the thousands of experiences shared together and the wishes, dreams, hopes, and fears of the parent and child and 2) the real day-to-day relationship that continues to unfold into the present. A parent's marriage may appear to change the way in which a parent will interact in the present or may even threaten to change how a parent views his or her child. Although you may have a sense that "everything has changed," you, as an adult, have the resiliency to retain your sense of self despite many changes that may (or may not) come along as a result of your parent's marriage. Some of the anxiety you may feel stems from a sense that the parent-child relationship is ending. Whether you have wished for a better relationship with a parent or to hold on to the relationship you have, you may feel that such wishes have been forever dashed. However, a parent's marriage may open new opportunities for growth for both you and your parent, if you are open to the possibility of such growth. Eric was able to take pleasure in the positive changes in his father's temperament rather than hold on to old grievances and, in so doing, found a connection that had long eluded them both.

Eric was a 45-year-old married father of three when his own 80-year-old father married after being a widow for 5 or 6 years. Eric had a distant relationship with his father since childhood despite his ardent wish for a closer relationship. When Eric was a boy, his father had been "too tired to play catch and too disinterested to watch me play Little League." As Eric grew into a man, the lack of involvement between him and his father continued. "He was always too busy, too tired, too grouchy, or just not there. I remember him most as someone I was more than a little frightened of. I was never close to him. I really never remember him being there for me either as a kid or even when I was older and just wanted to share interests in sports with him."

Eric's father married a woman who had been a reporter for a small-town newspaper, reporting of all things, the sports news! When Eric met his father and his new "bride" shortly after their wedding, Eric was stunned at the change in his father: "He was sporting a little goatee, and he just laughed all evening. I sat and watched my father and was simply amazed. For the next 3 years, I was able to have a relationship with my father that I had given up wishing for."

Your Parent's Marriage as
Violating the Natural Order of Life

Although life can throw you a curve ball from time to time, you probably realize that life is not one chaotic mass of random happenings; there is an order and organization to life. Humans operate according to a loosely drawn developmental plan that is more or less common to all: children grow up and become adolescents and then young adults; young adults go out into the world of college or work, socialize, and eventually pair off into some kind of significant relationship; then, if they so choose, they have a family of their own. As these events happen in their life, their parents are continuing through their part of the life cycle: they grow older and grayer and continue in their chosen careers in the world or at home; they grow a bit older and grayer, perhaps become a bit infirm, retire from their careers, and possibly relocate; and then they become a bit older and grayer, possibly become ill, and ultimately die. That is the expectable nature of things. Even if we never think much about this course of events, we "know" this to be true and expect it to happen.

A parent's marriage that is out of sync with this "schedule of life" challenges our mostly deeply held expectations about the progression of life. This untimely event may seem to work against the natural order of things, turning back the clock and placing the parent at a different point in the life cycle from where he or she is expected to be. In fact, the marriage may place a parent at seemingly the same point in the life cycle as that parent's child! The experience may be comparable to a teenager's parents trying to act young; most teenagers are mortified when their parents adopt the clothes, language, or even music that belongs to the younger generation. A parent marrying and beginning a new family, perhaps even starting a new career or moving to a new location, may seem just as out of place. It is common for adult children to feel that their parent's marriage is "weird," "wrong," "out of step," or "time warped." Sara, a 23-year-old graduate student, put it succinctly:

> It's weird to think about your parent getting married. I know a lot of people say "remarried," but it's still the same thing. It's just wrong somehow—not in any moral sense, but it just feels wrong.

Sometimes weddings just seem strange. Betty's mother married when Betty was age 42. Both Betty's mother and new husband had been widowed and had known each other casually through church activities. They were married in a church, and Betty could only recall an eerie feeling of strangeness settling over her as she watched her mother take her wedding vows. This "eerie" or strange feeling may have come from Betty's discomfort at watching something that emotionally feels as though it should have predated her existence.

An adult may unconsciously feel that he or she is intruding on a parent's space, seeing something that is forbidden by chronology, something that just can't be happening in an emotional world where parents marry before a child exists. And so, Betty and others like her who feel strange or weird at their parents' marriages may be reacting to this sense of time out of order, feeling like they are witnessing something that they cannot really witness!

★   Examine the issue of your parent's marriage being out of sync with the natural order of things. Take a paper and pen (or typewriter or computer), and list the reasons that your parent getting married makes sense. If your parent was already married, it may help to think about your parent as marrying again. If your parent has never been married, it may help to think about your parent's reasons for marrying now. Being able to look at your parent's marriage in the light of the present may help flush out any buried feelings that are making you feel strange and help you focus on the current reality of your parent's marriage, which is more than likely far less threatening or strange than anything clunking around in your unconscious.

★ Chapter 3 ★

If You Don't Like Your Parent's Spouse: Reasons You May Not Expect

Questions to Think About as You Read This Chapter

- Why don't you like your parent's choice for a spouse?
- Is it possible that, over the years, you have begun to fill a place in your parent's life that was more appropriately filled by a spouse? On some level, have you missed that child-parent relationship that has been slowly supplanted?
- How do your parent's actions reflect on your gender as a whole?

If you have decided you do not like your parent's choice for a spouse, you probably have your reasons all set out. They may be similar to those expressed by other adult children in the same situation as yourself:

- He is just different from the rest of our family. He is [pick one] less sophisticated/less educated/less monied.
- She is 3 years younger than myself; she's too young for him!

- She's an intellectual snob who is vulgar; not a bad person, just one who rubs you the wrong way.
- He's a fanatic about his religion. [Or the opposite:] She doesn't seem to believe in anything.
- She's of medium height, fat, with large bovine facial features and a personality to match.
- He's a used car salesman, one of the bad kind. He's not a pleasing or trustworthy person.
- He's ignorant, selfish, very forgetful, and abusive and has a bad temper.

The list could go on forever. However, underneath these "reasons" that your parent's spouse or intended spouse is not acceptable to you may lie the real reason you cannot accept him or her: your parent's relationship with this new person is threatening to you in some way. In the following sections, I explore how this could be the case.

You and Your Opposite-Sex Parent: Breaking Up Your "First Couple" . . . Again

Children's first relationship with a person of the opposite sex is typically played out between themselves and one of their parents. The sight of a small boy offering a handful of wildflowers—roots and all—to his mother, or a little girl looking up into her father's eyes, is often seen in greeting cards and television commercials because we were all once there, adoring our mothers or fathers . . . or wanting to. The relationship between ourselves and our opposite-sex parent remains powerful regardless of the actual quality of the original relationship.

At about age 3 years, during what is well known as the *oedipal period,* an intense struggle begins between a child's emerging sexuality and his or her same-sex parent for the affections of the opposite-sex parent. During this period, the evolving child develops in two important ways: 1) the child begins to form a gender identity (that is, a sense of being male or female) by comparing himself or herself with his or her parents, discerning the similarities to the same-sex parent and the differences from the opposite-sex parent, and 2) the child develops strong feelings for his or her parents. A parent's marriage may trigger old themes of identity and competition with the same-sex parent and with the oppo-

site-sex parent in various combinations. Although developmental paren-
theses are placed around such identity development, the feelings that
such growth evokes may be reconciled along the way to adulthood but
never put away forever.

Adults who have felt either too close to or too distant from their
opposite-sex parent may react strongly to that parent's marriage. It is
important to realize that these feelings may come as a surprise to the
adult child: If the child and parent have had a close relationship, then
the adult child might feel confused as to why he or she is not happy for
his or her parent. If the child and parent have had a distant relationship,
then such strong feelings might seem totally unexpected; feelings of jealousy and betrayal may be masked as embarrassment, disgust, or anger.

In the following sections, I explore the reactions adult children may
have when either their same-sex or their opposite-sex parent marries.

Sons and Mothers

Bill remembered the circumstances of his parents' divorce well:

> It was the summer that I graduated from college. I had planned to go
> away to law school. This was a very big deal in my family.
>
> I remember my parents went out to dinner about a week after my
> graduation. I had been home that evening as my mother was getting
> ready to go out. It's funny, but I still remember the dress she wore. It was
> some black thing, and I remember thinking that she looked good "for
> her age." When I think back and realize she wasn't even 40, I have to
> laugh at that statement. But anyway, I remember she was very happy that
> night—my father had called from the office and asked my mother to
> meet him at her favorite restaurant. It wasn't their anniversary or either
> of their birthdays or anything, and it was in the middle of the week so
> she was surprised. Well, she certainly was surprised: my father took her
> out, ordered wine and dinner, and then told her he wanted a divorce.
> I remember feeling so angry at him, so let down and disappointed. Of
> course, my first reaction was to tell my mother that I wouldn't be going
> away to school, that I would get a job and think about law school later
> on. Of course, she didn't let me. But, I remember that from that night
> on, I felt responsible for her. It was as though my father just handed her
> off to me.
>
> I called her every night from school for my entire first year. Most of
> the time, I could tell she had been crying; sometimes she started crying

while we were on the phone. I thought it was just the dirtiest trick that my father could have ever played on me. Of course, as I matured I realized that he had thought this was a good time, with my beginning law school, but actually somehow that made it worse. It was as though he had thought our whole life together as a family was just somehow ended when I was ready to begin my adult life. Did he really expect that my feelings for my mother would just evaporate because I was going away to school? I don't really know.

He got married as soon as the divorce was final; at least I didn't have to worry about any wedding. They took a trip to the Virgin Islands and came back and announced their marriage. Frankly, it never seemed quite real to me.

However, it was my mother's marriage that really got to me, because I never saw it coming. She had been divorced for 15 years. She had made a life for herself, as she liked to call it—she had a nice job in a quiet community, a condominium in her own name, a good settlement bringing in interest, and here and there a dinner engagement with, as she called him, "no one in particular." Well, about 2 years after my son was born, Mom called up and said that she wanted to come over and share some news. Then she dropped the bombshell that she and "no one in particular" were getting married; they were planning a small wedding and everything.

I was surprised at my reaction. Of course, I was polite to my mother, but I was seething inside. How after all these years of my taking care of her could she turn around and do this? I was humiliated. It was just ridiculous.

To understand a son's reaction to his mother's marriage, the son-mother relationship must be considered. After a father has left the family (whether through divorce, abandonment, or death), sons often place themselves in the position of being their mothers' protectors and champions, even though this is not a role they may actually want for themselves; rather, it is a role they feel has been forced on them by their departed fathers. In cases in which the mother is a widow, these feelings may be even more intensified. Then, when the mother decides to marry, the son perceives this as a "thanks, but no thanks," to which he reacts with otherwise unexplained anger. Of course, this anger is often channeled directly toward his mother's intended spouse. On some level, those ancient oedipal conflicts are being dragged out and enlivened (for example, the son feels himself in competition for his mother's affection), with the new added twist that the son feels as though "all he has done" is being belittled and discarded. Bill (above story) continued to call his mother's intended "Mr. No One in Particular" in a half-joking way until his mother, sensing the underlying hostility, asked him to stop.

Combined with this sense of no longer being needed can be a son's feelings of jealousy toward his mother's chosen partner. This may be expressed as his feeling that the intended is not good enough for his mother—which recalls the son's need to act as his mother's protector and save her from making a mistake; in reality, his feelings are based on jealousy. Jim found himself experiencing such feelings without realizing it:

> When my mother first decided to marry, I thought it wasn't a bad idea. I mean, it wasn't like she was an old lady or something, and I thought it would be a good idea for her to have company. But, this guy is a real dork. I mean he is a Class A jerk; I don't know what my mother sees in him. He has an okay job and everything, but you should just see him, and you'd know what I mean. Even the way he dresses! Now, I don't usually notice something like that in a guy, but this guy just stands out!

The embarrassment that many men feel when their mothers announce marital plans is an embarrassment that has its roots in the distant past. Remember Bill reminiscing about his mother and how she looked good the night she went to dinner with his father; now, the presence of another man in his mother's life—a man who is not his father—is a clear indication of his mother as a woman with her own sexuality. It is this embarrassment that may be working underneath many sons' claims of their mothers' unseemly, immature, silly, or otherwise unacceptable behavior. Actually, their own firmly buried conflicts about their mothers are calling up this embarrassment more than anything the mothers may or may not be doing.

Daughters and Fathers

Whereas sons are generally polite to their mothers when the subject of marriage is approached, daughters are generally quite vocal with their fathers.

> Carolyn was 30 years old and the mother of two small children when her parents divorced. As a young career woman, she was busy most of the

week but never too busy to call her father from the office, receive his phone calls to her, or even meet him for lunch once a month.

Carolyn felt that the divorce had left her father distraught; she saw her mother, with whom she maintained a relationship, as being more than a little selfish. "Whether he was on the phone or knocking on our door on a Sunday morning with the papers, I knew that Dad was lonely. Even though I had a very busy life at that stage, I was never too busy for Dad. Never. And then after 2 years of all these phone calls, lunches, and Sunday morning visits, he lowered the boom. It seems that he had fallen in love with someone who 'makes him feel like a youngster' and that he was getting married. I remember thinking that, when he told me she made him feel like a youngster, that he always was really immature. I couldn't believe that he was serious."

As Carolyn questioned her father intensely about his new relationship, she became concerned about his choice for a number of reasons, and vociferously expressed her concerns to him. She eventually realized that she was reacting based on her feeling of intense anger, masked as her concern for her father and her need to denigrate his choice. As she expressed it, "The strange part is, I didn't even really know with whom or about what I was angry. I was just consumed with anger."

In Francine's case, the overriding emotion in her reaction to her father's impending marriage was jealousy:

Father has been living alone for almost 8 years now. He was married for 2 years after my mother died, but that didn't work out, and he realized it quickly. He met this woman, Emily, at the movies one night. In fact, we were all there. He always sits in the back of the theater because he says we sit too close. Anyway, Emily was there with a friend sitting in the back row too, and they simply "struck up a conversation." Those are Emily's words, and if I hear them again, I think I'll scream. That's just an example, but you can get the idea; people never just talk in Emily's world or say anything; they "strike up conversations," they "respond," and so on and so on. I've never known such a boring person in my entire life! I usually can find something to like in anyone, especially another woman, but Emily? I'm still looking, but I can't find anything the least bit interesting!

Daughters have typically found themselves (or perhaps wished themselves to be) in the role of confidante for their fathers. They have realized their wish to "have their fathers" all to themselves with the dissolution of their parents' union by death, divorce, or abandonment. Regardless of whether they actually lived out this role of the "other woman" in their fathers' lives, many women with intense reactions to their fathers' marriages clearly feel "displaced" by their fathers' new partners. In the above examples, Carolyn was "never too busy to call her father from the office," and Francine was annoyed at the use of the phrase "strike up a conversation," as though anyone could just take her place and talk to her father. Both women clearly saw themselves as their fathers' protectors and listening ears, and both daughters in these examples clearly felt that they were superior to the other women in their fathers' lives. Carolyn felt that her mother was "selfish," and Francine stated that her father had "realized quickly" that his first marriage after her mother's death would not "work out." Both daughters felt that their special role had been usurped by the new women in their fathers' lives and, as such, reacted with intense anger.

You and Your Same-Sex Parent

Given the importance of your parents in the development of your gender identity, when your same-sex parent marries, you may experience powerful feelings of competition. The competition of a long-gone era may be rekindled in the present, but with a decidedly different twist. At ages 3–5, you were at a distinct disadvantage in your competition between yourself and your same-sex parent for the affections of your opposite-sex parent. Now, as an adult, the battle is similar, but you are grown and able to match wits in this competition because of your similar capacities for thinking and communicating your thoughts; you can play out long-ago rageful feelings of competition as an equal combatant. Furthermore, as an adult, you may still "want" your opposite-sex parent, but it is now clear that you do not "need" the same-sex parent to ensure your physical or psychological survival. The sense of standing on equal (or even superior) footing with the same-sex parent may translate into ridicule of the parent's relationship. Such feelings may be thinly masked behind descriptors of the new partner or the relationship as "ridiculous," "childish," and "foolish." Under the surface are feelings that seem just this side of downright hostile. In fact, adult children may be surprised at the intensity of this current of feeling and may begin to question even a previously stable working relationship with their parents.

Sons and Fathers

In general, sons give less importance to their fathers' marriages than do daughters. However, some painful issues may arise in the context of a father's marriage. Typically, sons learn their first concepts of being male from their fathers. Some men react with anger to their fathers' marriages. Again, this may hark back to that time long ago when a little boy felt he had to compete with his father for his mother's attention, but there are here-and-now considerations as well. Some men seem to resent their fathers' marriages, seeming to construe them as the means by which their fathers take something away from either their mothers (whether divorced or deceased) or—and this may be much harder to admit—themselves. If the son and father had a good relationship prior to the father's marriage, then the marriage generally does not present any significant problems for the son. In fact, sons who have had strong relationships with their fathers may fear that they are in danger of losing their fathers if the fathers have been unhappy or lonely living alone. Many men rely on their wives to foster social relationships, even extending to family visits, and fathers who are living alone often appear to withdraw from relationships. For this reason, sons may welcome their fathers' marriages, believing their fathers' renewed happiness would mean a return of their former good relations, as did Lou:

> Lou, who felt a deep love for his father, was happy when his father married 4 years after Lou's mother died. He explained his feelings as follows: "Dad had spent 3 years nursing my mother. His dedication to her was something I'll never forget. He seemed to take her death so personally. I really never thought I'd see him smile again. I can't tell you how it makes me feel to hear him laugh out loud again. I just know my mother is smiling too!"

However, if the father-son relationship was troubled before the marriage, then the marriage might be used as a scapegoat for problems that actually predated it. In particular, men whose fathers did not live with them during childhood may have a more difficult time adjusting than men who did spend time with their fathers throughout their lives. For example, Jon's father had had a series of relationships with women for as long as Jon could remember. He related this story:

My parents were divorced when I was about age 3, so I really don't ever remember them as a couple or us as a family. My father was only 27 years old or so when he and my mother were divorced, so there were always women in his life. He never seemed to have any really serious relationships. They'd be around for 1, 2, or 3 months, and then someone new would be introduced and that was that—until last spring. Out of the blue my father introduces me to this woman. She shows me her finger and there is this "rock" sitting on it. "We're engaged!" she says. I'm still not sure exactly why it hit me so hard, but it did.

In Jon's case, the only thing he apparently could count on with his father was his inability to form attachments to others. Jon had more than likely rationalized his father's "leaving" him as being in line with his father's inability to stay with anyone. However, when Jon's father became engaged, this defense was challenged, leaving Jon awash in feelings of loss and abandonment.

Another common reaction is embarrassment that the father may be being made a fool of.

Richard, a 35-year-old married man with three young children, greeted the idea of his father's marriage to a younger woman with unconcealed scorn. "My father is almost 70 years old, and here he is going around with a woman whom I could be marrying. She's clearly more in my age bracket than his. Maybe other people could just go on with this charade, but I don't care if he's hurt a little bit now. He'll thank me for it later, that I tried to stop him from making a fool of himself."

The elements of competition are heard clearly in this case. The parent's marriage calls into question the adult child's feelings of self. Listen carefully and you'll hear the old echoes of parental words in the adult child's feelings today. Ridiculous? Childish? A fool? The adult children have in their own emotions become the parents of yesterday. Now it is the parents who are being chastised for overstepping boundaries, risking ridicule by others who watch them. The feelings the adult child may be identifying in his or her parent are those same feelings the adult child felt all those years ago when he or she was in love with the very first person he or she knew who was different from himself or herself—the opposite-sex parent—and reacting against those feelings in his or her parent.

Daughters and Mothers

Daughters must struggle with some of the same issues with regard to their mothers' marriages as do sons with regard to their fathers' marriages. If a mother's marriage is "for love," those same troubling, age-old conflicts may surface. A daughter who is struggling with feelings of competition with her mother may describe her mother's impending partner as disgusting, repulsive, or horrible. Certainly it is possible that a mother's intended spouse is unappealing to the daughter; however, when pushed for an explanation, the daughter's responses often seem out of proportion to the described offenses. Linda, for example, "hates" her mother's husband because "he wears plaid shorts with a striped shirt"; Carla has similar negative sentiments toward her mother's husband because "he chews with his mouth open"; and Lydia "can't stand" her mother's husband "because he smells like cheap aftershave."

A daughter's reaction to her mother's marriage may also be derived somewhat from cultural expectations. For example, if a daughter expects that her mother should be able to be self-sufficient, then she will dismiss her mother's marrying as her mother's way of ensuring that there is someone there to take care of her. On the other hand, if a daughter believes that her mother must be taken care of, she may see the impending marriage in a more positive light.

Finally, it must be remembered that a woman learns her concept of femaleness first from her mother. A daughter may feel a personal stake in her mother's decision to marry, and her reasons for it may seem tied up with who she is as a woman. This may be especially true when a woman identifies particularly closely with her mother, as does Victoria:

> Victoria, a strikingly beautiful young woman, shows a picture of her mother, a very attractive woman who looks years younger than her age of 49 years. Victoria was 28 when her mother announced that she was planning to marry a man she had been dating for the past 2 years. Victoria had always prided herself on her good relationship with her mother, saying, "Why, she's like my best friend. In fact, she is my best friend. I could always tell her anything. Maybe it's because I grew up in the house alone with her. My father left when I was not quite 2 years old, and I really don't remember him. It was always Mom and me. But, I have to be honest, I just couldn't believe it when she said she was getting married. I mean it was so ridiculous, I just wanted to laugh. What does

she have to get married for? Is she planning on having more children? Raise another family? I can't believe her sometimes, maybe she just doesn't realize that there's really no need for her to get married at her age. I always thought we were so close. I thought I understood my mother better than anyone. But, I just don't understand this. I could understand her wanting a little companionship—but marriage at her age? I just don't get it. Honestly, it seems a little childish to me."

In the above example, Victoria has clearly borrowed her female identity from her mother and supplied for herself and her mother the father who was clearly always missing from the picture. These two women, almost mirror images of each other, may have functioned a bit like Narcissus, that is, very much in love with their own images reflected in each other. For Victoria, the notion that her mother planned to take on another and different object for her love may feel like a deep wound. To deal with this pain, Victoria seeks to denounce her mother, and thereby lessen the power of the wound, by reducing her mother's plans to little more than a childish whim. By reducing her mother's intentions in this way, she can, for a while, continue the fantasy that they do not need anyone else.

Chapter 4

Feeling Discarded: When Your Parent No Longer Seems to Need You

Questions to Think About as You Read This Chapter

- What role have you played in your parent's life during the past several years? In what ways is this role similar to or different from the role you have always played in your parent's life? Would you like your role in your parent's life to be different?
- Are you secretly relieved that some of the responsibility for caring for your parent will be lifted from you? Are you jealous that some of the responsibility for caring for your parent will now be shared?
- Do you have mixed feelings about the way in which your relationship with your parent will change now that he or she will be married? Have you discussed and defined these changes with your parent or simply made assumptions about them?
- Is there any possibility that you have been using your responsibilities toward your parent as a way of avoiding issues in your own life?

Your Relationship With Your Parent Since He or She Became a Single Parent

After parents separate, whether through divorce or death, their relationship with their adult children often changes: the newly single parent, once the protector and provider, becomes the protected and the recipient of help, and the adult child becomes the protector and provider of help. Long-married parents especially may have difficulty adjusting to a life in which they are no longer part of a married couple; to cope, they may begin to replace the interdependence of marriage with dependence on their children. In addition, single parents with grown children may feel their aloneness more keenly, fearing that they will live out the rest of their lives alone; to combat this fear, they may seek a more active role in their grown children's lives.

Relationships between adult children and single parents clearly vary with the individuals and circumstances involved, yet there are patterns to this help-giving and -receiving situation. Once your parent began living alone, you and your siblings probably experienced shifts in your roles and responsibilities toward your parent (e.g., increased phone calls, increased visits), whether he or she was living in the same town or across the globe. You may have been expected to assume a more supportive role for your parent at a time when you were just building or already involved in a life of your own with your own increasing responsibilities. For this shift in relationship to work, both child and parent must accept this new dependence, which can be difficult for both adult children and parents.

Parents Who Reach Out—Endlessly

Some parents seem to have no difficulty reaching out to their adult children. Their needs may seem to be insatiable; they are like hungry infants with a bottomless hunger. Parents who are so demanding are actually terribly needy. Just as children call on their mother again and again until they are sure of her reliability, parents now call on their children until they feel reassured by their children's constancy.

Adult children may attempt to meet these never-ending demands until they reach the point of saturation. Then they may try to avoid the onslaught of demands by handing off the responsibility to another family member or even to their own spouse.

Tom began to rue the day when he told his mother "call me whenever you need me." The first several times Tom's mother telephoned him at the office, she apologized for disturbing his workday, and he was quick to allay her concern. Her problems really never took up very much time, and she seemed to be so comforted by the solutions that he was able to offer. The calls at home—during dinner, before her bedtime, and sometimes later at night when she couldn't fall asleep or had just thought about something she wanted to share—quickly became irritating. After a few months, Tom was ashamed to admit that he had asked his secretary to screen his mother's calls at work, and his wife and three children did so at home. "Find out if it's an emergency" became his standard response.

> ★   Assure your parent that you will be available if you are actually needed rather than showing him or her that you are available by attempting to meet every small demand.

Parents Who Need Help and Refuse to Ask

The opposite of needy parents are those who are in obvious need but refuse to ask for help. These parents may not go to the store to buy things they would like to have or may miss important appointments because of transportation difficulties. Such parents can cause their adult children considerable anxiety.

Denise visited her mother one Sunday and noticed that her mother seemed to be having trouble chewing. When she asked her mother if everything was all right, Denise's mother finally admitted that she had missed several periodontist appointments because she had had a "falling out" with the friend who used to drive her. When Denise asked why her mother had not told her about her transportation problem, her mother would only reply, "I didn't want to bother you."

A parent who needs but does not ask for help may be afraid that if he or she overburdens the child, the request will be rejected. The potential of such rejection may raise issues for the parent of being left and exacerbate his or her sense of vulnerability and loneliness. The person then who is "not bothered" is the parent, who in being able to shelve his or her obvious need for assistance can only shelve the anxiety about needing someone else that, for him or her, comes with such a request. One way to decrease a parent's discomfort in asking for help is to clearly let a parent know that although you may not be personally able to do the task for the parent, you will help your parent get things done. Emphasize to a parent the attitude of "teamwork" by perhaps offering examples from your own life about how you get things done with the cooperation of others. By offering your life as an example, parents may begin to change their perception of "asking for help" to an opportunity to brainstorm to get things done. In this way, parents do not have to feel infantilized or any tinge of uncomfortable role reversal, and adult children will minimize the risk of feeling on edge.

The social mores operative when parents were raised will affect their perception of the degree to which they can comfortably seek help. For example, women of an earlier generation would most likely find it easier to ask for help than would men of the same generation, who were raised to be self-reliant.

> ★ Encourage your parent to keep a "things that need to be done" list, which you can then look at together.

Your Relationship With Your Parent After His or Her Marriage

When your parent marries, you may find that the roles you and your parent are accustomed to playing are suddenly recast. Your parent is once again a husband or wife, you are now someone else's stepchild, and, if there are children from this new marriage, you may have stepsiblings along with a whole crowd of other "instant relatives." Also, as someone who has been accustomed to relating to your parent as a solitary unit, you will have undoubtedly formed certain expectations about your and your parent's future that did not include this cast of characters. You may find that you lose certain roles in your parent's life or take on additional roles with regard to your parent and his or her new spouse.

Role of Caregiver

One role that is common to adult children of single parents is that of caregiver (for example, running errands for the parent, driving a parent to appointments), although sons and daughters appear to perceive these responsibilities in a different light. In addition to the errands, daughters often give more emotional support to the parent in terms of making and receiving telephone calls, listening to complaints and fears, and sharing the parent's joys and disappointments. On the other hand, sons more typically feel that caregiving for an adult parent has been completed once an errand has been run or financial responsibility has been taken or if the task has been successfully assigned to another. These generalizations may be losing their validity, as men are becoming more inclined to discuss feelings with their parents. But for now, it seems that the bulk of emotional support for single parents is taken up by daughters rather than sons.

The differences in the ways in which sons and daughters typically interact with their parents may influence how they handle their parents' marriage and new spouse. For example, sons tend to be more practical in their concerns about their parents' marriage, viewing marriage as an arrangement rather than a romance. Daughters, on the other hand, view the marriage as a love connection.

Being Displaced as Your Parent's Caregiver

Feeling cheated.   Some adult children feel displaced—thrown out—and replaced by a stranger who will now take care of their parent, a role that they themselves had expected to fulfill. Samantha was one such woman:

> Samantha and her husband had already talked about the possibility that her mother, who had been widowed 3 years previously, would move into their large suburban home, even though her mother was only 38 years old. Samantha was sure that her mother would want to be close to her three grandchildren and be "right there on the scene" for their school plays, games, graduations, and parties. As she explained it, "I remember how much Mom enjoyed that when my sister and I were children, and I just knew she would want to be a large part of the girls' lives"—or so she thought.
>
> Although Samantha was not certain how she would feel about hav-

ing her mother living in her home, she was sure that if the right guide-lines were set at the outset in terms of boundaries and friends visiting and so forth, that it would probably work out. Her husband, Tim, was not so sure. Samantha reminisced, "I remember Tim saying that Mom was still young and that maybe she would meet someone. Now I have to laugh thinking about how angry I got at the very idea and how right Tim was after all." Before Samantha could even mention the idea of her mother moving in, her mother introduced Bill to the family at a Christmas party, and on New Year's Eve she called to announce her engagement.

Samantha described the anger this announcement engendered in her: "It may sound silly, but I just felt so annoyed—like I had gone to all this trouble, put myself through so much in coming to terms with accepting her as part of my family because, frankly, I didn't think there was any other option. Now that I think of it, I just always expected somewhere deep down that I would take care of her the way she took care of me."

Sons can feel the same sense of betrayal and of being deprived of some undefined expected responsibility, as did Frank:

Frank was in his first year of medical school when his father, the founder of a large locally based company, suddenly died. The older of two sons, Frank left medical school, completed an MBA, and became an active member in the family business along with his mother.

Within 3 years of his father's death, Frank's mother announced her engagement to an old family friend. Frank described his reaction: "I felt an incredible sense of betrayal and, yes, anger. I had changed my entire life around for the family and now this! It was as though my mother and this man were just wiping out my life along with my father's. It was an extraordinarily powerful and painful time for me."

In listening to Samantha and Frank, you can hear the sense of loss in being deprived of something. The relationship between a parent and an adult child is very complex, woven from the threads of a lifetime of memories, hopes, and expectations. An adult child may put his or her parent on the adult child's timetable of expectations without realizing it: expecting the parent to retire, perhaps relocate to a new senior commu-nity, or do a bit of traveling. A marriage by a parent may throw this timetable off and leave the adult child feeling vaguely cheated.

Samantha's and Frank's sense of deprivation revolves around the loss of yet another expectation: the expectation that, all things being normal, they would eventually complete the life cycle and be expected to take care of their parents as their parents once took care of them. A parent's remarriage, therefore, is seen as depriving them of the obligation to take care of their parents. Adult children may feel cheated out of showing their parents what a good job they could do. They may have unconsciously looked forward to the time when they could be the boss and not only demonstrate their competence to their parents but also completely reverse that old power imbalance between parent and child.

★ Do not assume that your relationship with your parent will change on the basis of his or her marriage.

★ To reduce your concerns and any possible confusion, discuss with your parent the ways in which your relationship with and responsibilities for him or her will change.

★ Accept the idea that some of the responsibility for caring for your parent will now be shared with another.

Feeling relieved.   If you have been taking care of your parent before your parent decided to marry, then you may feel relieved at your parent's decision. This is okay. Many adult children secretly feel guilty over their relief and work against themselves by trying to continue caregiving that is no longer wanted or required by either their parents or the new spouse. So, if your parent can now manage with less help from you, enjoy the new arrangement.

Taking on a double burden.   Sometimes a parent marries someone who is not accustomed to looking after himself or herself. In that case, if an adult child has already been taking care of his or her parent, then the new spouse may come to expect to be taken care of as well. In this case, the adult child may come to resent the new spouse and these added demands. It is important to get additional help when the caregiving burden increases. An adult child may help his or her parent help the new spouse to secure help from the spouse's family or from private or, if applicable, social services. On the other hand, an adult child who has become accustomed to doing a good deal of caregiving may feel a sense of relief because he or she can continue in this same role as caregiver.

Feeling Guilty About Not Having Been a Good Caregiver

For adults who have not been involved in a great deal of caregiving for their parents—perhaps because they live far away, or they have maintained an independent relationship with their parents—when their parents decide to marry, they may experience an odd feeling of loss and a niggling sense of guilt at not having been more involved. Suzanne, age 46 years, reflects on this sense of not having done enough:

> It was strange. I was always proud of my mother and my relationship with her. Mother had been a career woman as I am, and when she retired, she just kept on going—continuing to socialize with friends she had had for a lifetime and making new friends through the new activities she acquired. Both she and I had a full life of activity and people we enjoyed spending time with. She substituted her work life with a full schedule of volunteer work, and I, of course, continued to work. I don't think it would have ever occurred to either my mother or myself that I should be taking care of her. I'm sure both of us would have laughed off the suggestion; in fact, my mother probably would have resented the suggestion. Yet when my mother told me that she was getting married and she wouldn't have to be alone anymore, I was stunned. I really felt that I had let her down in some monumental way.

Emptying the Nest . . . Again

For adults with grown or almost grown children, a parent's marriage can signify yet another loss. Many adults "feather their empty nests" with parental demands. Providing a sympathetic ear for parents, making phone calls to check on a parent, and taking a parent to doctor and dental appointments, for haircuts, and on shopping trips are all ways in which adult children spend time looking after their parents. Much of the errand running and caregiving is reminiscent of the adult child's activities in raising his or her own children. As much as adults may gripe and complain about how much of their time their parent consumes, you can be sure that along with the resentment is a parallel feeling of being needed—a feeling that may not be acknowledged until a parent announces his or her intention to marry. Then, strange feelings of loss wash over the adult child.

★ Use some of your "extra" time to refocus on your own life.

★ Decide what role you would like to have in your parent's life, then take an active part in making that happen. Speak to your parent and his or her spouse about your expectations, and negotiate any problem areas.

Chapter 5

Here Comes the Bride:
You and Your Parent's Wedding Day

Questions to Think About as You Read This Chapter:

- To what extent does your parent want you to be involved with his or her wedding—either planning it, participating in it, or both? How much do you want to be involved in the wedding?
- If you don't want to be involved but your parent wishes you to be, what are your reasons for not wanting to be?
- If you do want to participate but your parent does not wish you to be involved, have you discussed your wishes with your parent?
- If, despite all your best efforts, your parent's and your wishes concerning your involvement in the wedding are not compatible, what will you do?
- If you are having a very difficult time imagining remaining polite and pleasant at the wedding, ask yourself why.

Seeing a parent marry can be a unique experience. It can be unsettling, poignant, even humorous, or a combination of all three. Regardless of how you feel, a parent's wedding will provide rich material for personal growth.

Even if you support and encourage your parent in his or her upcoming wedding, the practical considerations of the wedding may present a minefield of difficult decisions, ranging from wording of wedding announcements, to whom to invite, to what your role in the wedding should be. How you and your parent handle these tricky issues can reverberate throughout the nuclear and extended family for years to come. Here are some guidelines and food for thought on these questions.

Announcing the Engagement

Telling the Family

Before the news of an engagement is made public, it is important that your parent tell the immediate family members and others who might be directly affected by the engagement. Children of the bride and groom, regardless of age, should be told about the impending marriage directly by the parent who is going to be married—ideally without the affianced present. However, no matter how careful the parent is, the news of a marriage often comes as a surprise, as Suzanne experienced when she answered the phone sleepily late one night:

> "Guess what?" my mother said. I couldn't guess. I was trying to stop my heart from pounding by being woken up at 2:00 A.M. "Milt and I are getting married." All I could do was ask, "Who's Milt?"

Who Tells the Other Parent?

If your parents were divorced, the "chore" of telling your other parent about your parent's marriage may fall to you. If residual bad feelings persist between your two parents, keep the announcement of the news simple and to the point, saying

> "I have some news to tell you. Dad/Mom is getting married to _____ on _____."

In fact, whatever your original parents' relationship, your announcement will always be brief, for two simple reasons. First, if your mother and father have an amicable relationship, there will be no reason for you to be the one to elaborate, for presumably they have already talked together. On the other hand, if their relationship is not amicable, the less said the better. Under such circumstances, news of a parent's marriage will usually trigger a reaction from the other parent that ranges from being uninterested to feeling enraged.

Whether an adult child "should" be responsible for telling one parent about the marriage of the other parent may be besides the point. Many parents simply go their own ways after their divorce and have little or no contact with each other, although their children maintain contact. If this is so, the adult child will usually have a good deal of experience in informing one parent about important events in the other parent's life.

If, on the other hand, the separated parents have contact with each other, it is more appropriate to ask the parent if he or she wants to announce the news himself or herself before someone else announces the news. Indeed, even in the prior situation in which parents have had little or no contact, the adult child will be served well to ask the marrying parent about his or her wishes.

Under no circumstances should you become involved in bad-mouthing your soon-to-be married or recently married parent. Although siding with one parent against the other may feel good for the moment, this will not serve you well in the long run. Even if you have previously been drawn into battles between your parents, this news can be viewed as a good opportunity to step out of the middle.

Making the Formal Announcement

If you like, you and any of your adult siblings may announce your parent's engagement. A newspaper announcement might read as follows:

> The daughters of Mrs. John Doe [if a widow; use Mrs. Cynthia Doe if a divorcée] of Brookline, Massachusetts, have announced Mrs. Doe's engagement to. . . .

Invitations

If your parent decides to have a formal wedding, engraved invitations would be considered proper. The following are some suggested wordings for the invitation:

The honor of your presence
is requested
at the marriage of
Mrs. John Doe [if bride is a widow]
Mrs. Cynthia Doe [if bride is a divorcée]
to
Mr. Ted Smith....

An alternative might be:

Mrs. John Doe
and
Mr. Ted Smith
request the honor of your presence
at their marriage....

Bridal Showers and Parties

It is acceptable for a bride who has been married before to have a bridal shower or engagement party. If, as the child of either the bride or the groom, you want to host such a gathering, go right ahead. Even if you feel you were not informed about the decision to marry, or the marriage has already occurred, it will serve you well to have some sort of celebration for yourself, your parent, and his or her new spouse or spouse-to-be. This gathering may be as simple as a dinner in your own home or a local restaurant or as lavish as a catered affair in a private club. Your sponsoring of such a party would be your acknowledgment of your parent's decision to marry.

The Wedding Gown

Today it is acceptable for brides who have been married before to wear a wedding gown at their subsequent wedding. If your advice is asked, you may refer the bride to one of the many excellent etiquette books available today (see reference list), or you may simply help the bride to organize the kind of wedding she wants to have at this time of her life.

Many women may have had little control over the details of their first wedding, whereas they can have much more control over a wedding taking place later in their life. Therefore, a bride may choose to wear a traditional wedding gown at her second wedding to realize her long-held dream of having a wedding with all the trimmings, particularly if that was not the case for the first wedding. Try to be a good sport, and try to avoid switching roles and becoming a harsh, judgmental parent. Dr. Samuel Johnson (1769) quipped that "a second marriage is a testament of the triumph of hope over experience."

Participating as an Attendant in the Wedding

It is not uncommon for brides and grooms with adult children to ask their children to be attendants at the wedding. (As you read this section, keep in mind that many of the same issues occur if your children are asked to be in the wedding party [for example, as a ring bearer, a flower girl, or an usher].) If this occurs, treat the invitation with the respect it deserves. Whether you choose to accept or decline, this should be done in a polite manner.

Declining to Be an Attendant

If you are tempted to decline to be an attendant, think about why you are choosing not to participate. Remember that this is your parent's day and that you, along with all other invited guests, are being asked to simply witness—not approve—this event. If you feel you must decline, be courteous and sensitive; you do not need to share your personal travails over your decision at this time. If you clearly recognize that your objections to your parent's marriage are centered within yourself, you might simply let your parent know that you are still working out issues that are complicated for you but that do not affect your hope for their happiness. If you have serious objections to your parent's choice of partner and have stated these objections, you may have to simply agree to disagree.

What other possible motivations could be lurking behind such refusals? Are you somehow hoping to shock your parent into canceling the wedding by not participating, or do you want to hurt the parent now as perhaps you were once hurt yourself? If these feelings are truly intense and you cannot seem to deal with them, do not hesitate to seek some professional help. The marriage of a parent can be an excellent wellspring to thaw long-frozen feelings and perhaps finally free you to love your parent, yourself, and others more openly than ever before.

Be sure to think long and hard about your decision to decline being an attendant; once you have sorted out your feelings toward your parent's impending marriage, you may regret the decision not to participate in the wedding party. Remember that the wedding will take place regardless of whether you are an attendant. Furthermore, you may find that your feelings change with time. If you think there is even the slightest chance that you and your parent will continue to have a relationship after this wedding, rethink your decision to decline. Carin worked out her dilemma in the following way:

> My mother asked me to be her matron of honor, and I was floored. To tell the truth, I don't like the guy she is going to marry. I don't really think he's good enough for her. I know that probably a lot of people think that way about their mothers, but there are some strong differences in their backgrounds, and I just don't think they'll be happy. After I accepted to be her matron of honor, I was going to call her back and tell her I had changed my mind. Then a friend of mine called, and I started thinking and realized that if my friend were in the same situation but I thought she was making a mistake, I would still be in the wedding party. I realized that once my friend had made her decision to marry, I'd keep my mouth shut! I decided then and there that I'd try to treat my mother with the same respect as I'd treat a friend. If the marriage didn't work out, I'd be there for her, and I would never tell her I told you so!

- ★ Try thinking about your parent as a friend who is getting married and conduct yourself as you would with a friend who wanted (or did not want) your participation.
- ★ Imagine your parent's marriage lasting 20 or 30 years or more. Would you want to be remembered for the way you are planning on acting at the wedding?
- ★ Decide how you would act if you could be your own "ideal self," then imitate this behavior.

Accepting to Be an Attendant

Being asked and accepting to be an attendant can have many positive re-percussions in your parent's and your relationship. On your parent's side, asking you to be an attendant is one way in which he or she publicly acknowledges acceptance of you as an adult and as a very important part of his or her life. For the adult child, acting as a member of the wedding may encourage renewed feelings of bonding with the parent around this joyful event.

For many adults, a parent's marriage may be viewed as a renewed commitment to life, love, and joy and as a testament to the human spirit's capacity to reach out to another despite past hurt, disappointment, or grief. Being a formal witness to this act of human faith can be very in-spiring for the adult child as well as for the assembled guests who observe this union of family in happiness.

Even after accepting to be an attendant, some adult children still have mixed feelings about their role, as did Jack:

> Jack was asked and agreed to be his father's best man at his wedding to a very wealthy woman. Jack's father had owned a small business and had provided Jack and Jack's mother with a comfortable lifestyle. However, Jack was unprepared for the extent of the lavishness of his stepmother's townhouse. The wedding was a very formal affair, and Jack quickly felt completely out of place. Immediately, he realized that he would have been more comfortable if he could have acclimated to these heady sur-roundings by being a less visible participant in the wedding. However, he did not want to let his father down. Jack found his uneasiness growing throughout the wedding day as he increasingly felt that he, and his dis-comfort, were on display for all to see.

Jack's case shows how a new stepparent with a different lifestyle can, with or without intention, cause an adult child to feel different and, in some way, diminished. The disparity between the new lifestyle and the old can cause jarring comparisons and a sense of being alienated from the marrying parent. One clear way to avoid such situations is to learn as much as possible about the person whom your parent intends to marry and to remember that a parent's new style of living is not a judgment on a previous way of life.

Not Being Asked to Be an Attendant

Your parent is not obligated to ask either you or your children to be attendants. Your parent may feel that you and your children already play a significant part in his or her life and may prefer instead to be attended by peers.

To handle disappointing feelings generated by not being asked to be an attendant, try a simple method first: discuss your feelings with your parent. The parent may have been unsure about your desire to be a more active participant. However, if your parent does not wish to add you to the list of attendants, all is not lost. Rather than stewing in disappointed, hurt feelings, understand and become more proactive; being an attendant is far from the only way of feting a bride or groom!

> ★ If you want more involvement than you are being offered, consider hosting a dinner, luncheon, or other type of get-together (provided it does not conflict with other plans) that will permit you to get involved in wishing your parent and his or her new spouse well.

Guest List—What About Your Other Parent's Relatives?

The decision to invite or not to invite members of your other parent's family must be left to your parent and his or her intended spouse. Do not introduce yourself into or allow yourself to be cajoled into helping make decisions about who from your other parent's side of the family is to be invited. This is your parent's wedding and your parent's guest list.

Wedding Alternatives

Adults marrying for the second time, especially later in life, usually feel freer to deviate from "standards" regarding weddings. For example, years ago, if a wedding was anything but a first wedding, etiquette deemed it must be a quiet affair. Such ceremonies bore little resemblance to first weddings. Brides were not permitted to wear wedding gowns or to have attendants. The guest list was minimized to only the prerequisite legal witnesses, and if there was a celebration, it was very simple. Today, it is considered completely acceptable for individuals entering a second or subsequent marriage to celebrate their wedding along the lines of their first wedding.

Jennifer's mother and stepfather liked getting married so much, it appears, that they did it three times—marrying once in Arizona, once in Washington, D.C., and once in New York! In each location, they celebrated with different family members and friends. The problem for the family is that no one quite knows which anniversary to celebrate!

Gay Marriages

Stan's father called him to announce that he and his friend of 10 years, Daniel, were planning on marrying in a private ceremony. Although gay marriages are not legal in his state, Stan's father wanted Stan to attend the ceremony and share in his commitment to his lover. Felice's mother decided that she and her partner wanted to formalize their relationship and be recognized as a couple.

A parent's marriage to a same-sex partner may raise all of the same issues as those raised by an opposite-sex marriage and then some. It is especially helpful for the adult child to recognize that the ritual of a wedding ceremony is a public demonstration by two human beings of their joy, love, and commitment to each other. The religious or legal sanctions that are attendant to these functions are intended to support the solemnity of the commitment rather than create the commitment. Gay marriages are not legally recognized in most states; however, your parent is obviously motivated by a powerful desire for recognition as a couple. If you, as an adult child, are still having difficulty accepting the reality of a parent's sexuality, there may be no better wedding gift than working through such powerful issues with a professional trained in this specialized area.

Parents Who Elope

Although a parent's wedding often prompts a flood of challenges and concerns, the lack of a wedding is a problem too. Many older parents simply go off, marry, and then announce the accomplished fact to their children. Elopements seem to produce the same array of complicated emotions regardless of the age of the "elopees." Adult children may feel angry, hurt, rejected, or stunned—but they will probably feel alienated and unable to accept the fact of the marriage as a reality. When Helene's father surprised her with the news of his marriage, she had the following reaction:

> I just couldn't believe it. My father calls me on all special occasions, and when I heard his voice, I flipped through the calendar in my mind to see if I had forgotten anything. Well, it seems I hadn't; actually, I was being informed about a new special occasion to remember. What he actually said was, "Get out your calendar and mark down this day. I just got myself married." He was calling from Las Vegas. The whole thing just didn't seem real.

The rationale for weddings being public events was to inscribe the new union as a reality for those who witnessed its beginning. It is easier to dismiss something as less real if we have not actually seen it for ourselves. Moreover, an elopement deprives the adult child of sharing this important life experience with the parent and, in so doing, precludes the possibility of viewing the new spouse in the loving light of exchanged vows. Whereas a wedding can feel inclusive, an elopement may seem to imply that the adult child has no part in this new marriage.

Although you might be disappointed at being left out of your parent's wedding, you are free to arrange a celebratory event to mark the marriage. Whether a simple dinner at home or a formal party with invited guests, hosting such an event serves the important purpose of making this union real for you and for your family.

Adults Who Live Together but Remain Unmarried

Sometimes a parent decides to move in with someone without getting married. Senior citizens may decide to forgo marriage for financial reasons (for example, certain benefits may be cut if a person marries). For Tom, his mother's decision to share an apartment with her long-time companion had added benefits.

> When my mother said that she had something to tell me, I was at first worried about her health. She seemed so slow to get to the point, insist-

ing on making me a sandwich first and then a fresh pitcher of iced tea. When she finally got around to telling me that she and her friend were moving in together, I just about didn't hear her, and when I did, I couldn't believe it. Was this the same woman who practically stopped speaking to me when she found out my college girlfriend and I had shared the same room on spring break? I said something like that to her, and I re-member her answer to this very day: "But, Thomas dear, that was so very long ago!"

Sometimes we hold on to a parent's rigid viewpoints long after the parent's attitude has evolved. For Tom, understanding that his mother had grown and changed in many ways not only freed him from some long-standing guilt about his own "wild college days" but also allowed him to realize that human development is a continuing process. Never-theless, some adults may find that they disapprove of their parents' living situations. After such disapproval is voiced, it can certainly be held onto, but it is important for an adult child to accept that his or her role is not to approve or disapprove but simply to find a place for the parent in his or her own life.

★ **Chapter 6** ★

Is Your Parent Competent to Decide to Marry?

Questions to Think About as You Read This Chapter

- Do you feel that your parent is incompetent to make his or her own decisions?
- How long have you felt that your parent is incompetent? Why has this become a pressing issue now? Why have you never taken steps before?
- Are there other family members who agree with your assessment? If not, how is their opinion different?
- Have you stated or are you willing to state your concerns to an appropriate professional? If not, why not?
- Are you trying to use your parent's mental competence as an issue for a stopping a wedding you object to on other grounds?

In some cases, adult children may be concerned that their parents are incompetent to make decisions about their own lives, including the decision to marry. If your parent has decided to marry, but you are concerned about his or her mental competency to make that decision—especially if you feel that your parent would not make the same decision if he or she were competent—the only alternative for you is to consult with an attorney at once for the protection of your parent and his or her assets.

What Is Mental Incompetence?

Mental incompetence is a specific legal term that is used to determine whether a person is of "sound mind" as defined by law. The legal test of sanity or competency is whether a person's acts and conduct correspond with *that person's* normal acts and conduct. The way the law is written, competency or soundness of mind is not determined by comparison with that of the average "normal" person, because the law holds that no such measure of "normal" person exists. Instead, for the parent's acts to be judged sound, the acts and conduct under investigation must correspond with the acts and conduct of the parent at the time when he or she has been conceded to have been of sound mind. Note that procedures for legal recognition of marriage vary from state to state, but all states have minimum competency requirements.

A person can be judged incompetent only after he or she has been evaluated by a psychiatric professional, and a court has made a ruling to that effect based on the psychiatric evaluation and other relevant information. Usually signs of a person's incompetence will have been apparent for some time before reaching this legal stage. If a person is judged to be incompetent, he or she will be placed into the custody of another adult.

Incompetence is not to be taken lightly. It cannot be stressed enough that your disagreement over a decision your parent has made—including the decision to marry—does not indicate that that decision was an incompetent one. If your parent is not incompetent by the standards outlined above, do not attempt to have him or her so declared. Declaring a parent incompetent is a difficult process, both emotionally and practically, and should never be undertaken unless you are absolutely certain that it is in your parent's best interests. This was the case for Susan's mother:

> Susan's mother was given the diagnosis of early-stage Alzheimer's disease just after the beginning of the new year. Susan, her two brothers, and her sister felt that, because they all lived in the same city, they would be able

to care for their mother with a minimum of outside help. They were assured by their mother's physician that she did not yet require full-time supervision and that she could remain living in her own home for the time being.

Susan explained what happened next. "What we didn't expect was that around Valentine's Day Mother would announce that she had met a wonderful man who had delivered the flowers my brother had sent her. He was so wonderful that he had been coming around every evening to help her inventory her considerable collection of antique clocks and other expensive collectibles. We became even more alarmed when she had trouble remembering his name, seeing this as a sign of her beginning short-term memory loss."

Within about 2 weeks, this man began spending every day at the house after he got off work. By the beginning of spring, he announced to us that he was going to marry our mother and put an end to us snooping around her things! It broke our hearts, but we knew we had to do something.

Susan's mother's case was a rather straightforward case of a person becoming incompetent to make a responsible decision about marriage. Other cases are obviously more complicated. For example, if your parent decides to, as one woman put it, "throw all my money off the Empire State Building," that is your parent's decision. However, if your parent decides to throw all the money to the wind but a few minutes later asks you for an accounting of his or her funds, that is a different story.

★ Be very clear about the nature of your parent's incompetence. Are you concerned about a physical illness or disability or deterioration of mental processes?

★ Ask yourself, "Why now?" List your specific concerns and why they are an important issue at this time. When did you first notice your parent's incompetence?

★ Think about how this marriage will affect your parent's incompetence. See if others support your opinion.

★ Consult a professional in the appropriate field, get a second opinion, and then make a decision along with your other family members.

Foolishness or Incompetence?

If you think your parent is competent but acting perhaps "foolishly" in deciding to marry a certain individual, you might think about addressing the following questions: What is foolishness? What are your objections to foolishness in your parent?

For our purposes, let us assume that your definition of foolishness is not simply related to your sense of inappropriateness or embarrassment at your parent's choice of a partner but rather driven by a concern for his or her well-being. Some serious concerns might be that you believe an individual will mistreat your parent physically or that his or her claims of love and affection seem fraudulent. If you have examined your own motives, such as fear that you will lose an inheritance or your parent's affection, and still feel that your parent's judgment in this choice is poor, you can seek some professional help for yourself, with the goal of bringing your parent for joint counseling. If your parent agrees, then you will have an arena in which to discuss your concerns with a trained professional. On the other hand, if your parent refuses, then you will have found a safe haven in which you can air, learn to cope with, and/or resolve your concerns. You may also want to scan the bookshelves for titles that explain your point of view. Then, you must find a way to step back and let your parent have his or her own right to make his or her own mistakes, as you were (or wished you were) allowed to do by him or her!

★ **Section II** ★

You, Your Parent, and Your New Stepfamily

★ Chapter 7 ★

Adding a New Branch to the Family Tree

Questions to Think About as You Read This Chapter

- What kind of relationship would you like to have with your new stepparent? Is it different from or similar to what your parent and stepparent envision? Have you discussed your differences with them?
- What kind of relationship would you like to have with your other step-relations? Is it different from or similar to what your parent and stepparent envision? Again, have you discussed your differences with them?
- What actions have you taken to bring about the kind of relationship that you would feel most comfortable having with these new relations?
- If your parent and stepparent had a child together, do you ever think about your new half sister or half brother as a younger version of yourself? Do you watch your parent to see how he or she raises this child to learn more about the way in which you were raised? Do you compare the way you were raised with the way this child is raised?

When your parent marries, his or her new spouse may bring along a family of his or her own, to be integrated to some degree with your parent's family.

As your parent's child, you will be a part of that combined family, possibly with new stepsiblings, and certainly with a new stepparent.

The addition of a new stepparent can also have a ripple effect as you struggle to integrate his or her relatives, including brothers, sisters, children, and parents. If you are struggling with integrating just your parent's spouse into the family, this new crowd of people can be overwhelming—logistically and emotionally; indeed, it may feel like you are adding on an entire new limb to an already rooted family tree. If you have children of your own, you must decide how they will relate to their new uncles, aunts, cousins, grandparents, and so forth.

How do you negotiate your way through this new maze of relationships and role expectations?

A Replacement Family?

The expectation that this newly formed group of individuals can now act like a family may seem contradictory to you, given that families are usually identified by their shared history, traditions, and even objects. You may resist accepting your new family, feeling that your parent is trying to replace your original family with this new one; the situation may generate feelings of anger, anxiety, confusion, hurt, and sadness, among others. You can work your way through your emotional reaction by accepting the new family for what it really is: a new family that is an alternate—not a replacement—for your original family; this new family is a family to be enjoyed in the present.

Accepting a stepfamily can be especially difficult if the breakup of the original family left still-unhealed rifts. For example, even after his father had been married for 32 years to his second wife, Gerard still felt strongly negative toward his father's "new" family: "I don't know my stepmother's family at all, and I really don't care to."

The sense of the stepfamily being "his [the father's] family" and the original family remaining as "our mother's family" can be so strong that it is never overcome.

Thus, feelings among extended families can range from Bill's "Never met them, never wanted to" to Kim's "We are a family. We all get along just fine." When you get right down to it, there are as many variations in extended stepfamilies as there are in extended families.

In this chapter, I explore the relationship of an adult child with each type of new family member, one by one, to help guide you through the difficult process of adjusting to your new family.

Your New Stepparent

Sharing Your Parent

The issue that seems to be the main barrier between an adult child and his or her stepparent is the latter's perceived potential for intruding and perhaps irrevocably altering the parent–adult child relationship. Stepparents who are reported as the most loving and respected by their stepchildren are those who seem to be able to find a place for themselves in the family while understanding the need for closeness and even time alone between the parent and child. Stepparents who have the most conflicted relationships with their spouses' children seem to be those who are in some way threatened by the child's relationship with the parent and who let those fears guide their actions.

Some adult children relate that they have felt that their relationships with their parents were, in fact, interrupted by the new marriage. Given this understanding, many adult children long to hear their stepparents address this issue of interruption in the child-parent relationship, perhaps by making statements such as

- I am sorry for chasing you away.
- I will step back from your individual relationship with your father or mother.
- I will let the two of you work out any difficulties that arise between you without my interference (no matter how well intentioned I may think my involvement).

Sometimes a parent-child relationship is indeed lessened in intensity after a parent's marriage. All new marriages are typically self-involved, and it is not unusual for newly married people of any age to withdraw from others initially and devote much of their time to each other. It may be helpful to put off any decisions about how the parent-child relationship has changed until the marriage has had some time to grow roots of its own.

Sometimes family rifts are created as a result of tensions surrounding a stepparent's unresolved role in the family; both the parent and the adult child may long to heal those rifts but may not know how to begin that healing process.

> Jill and her father went to war over his intention to marry a woman whom Jill felt was very competitive and resentful of her relationship with her widowed dad. Jill felt that this new woman intruded on her relationship with her father, not understanding her continued need to have some time alone with him. Their difficulties eventually resulted in the father ostensibly siding with his new wife; following that break, Jill and her father ceased all contact with each other. Jill would love to hear her father say, "I love you and need you in my life. I don't want to grow old without you or without ever knowing my grandchildren."

Relationships cannot be mended unless someone gives in. In the above example, it seems that Jill very much wants to mend her relationship with her father, yet she is passively waiting for him to say the things she so very much wants to hear. Jill, and others like her who find themselves in broken relationships, might try taking a much more active role. For example, Jill might try *telling* her father just what she has waited so long for him to say to her: "I love you Dad and need you in my life. I don't want to grow older without you or without you ever knowing your grandchildren."

Many other issues can arise between parent and child over a stepparent:

> Harold, a 30-year-old machinist, has been struggling with his overbearing stepmother for 7 years. Harold's annoyance with his stepmother stems from the different way people do things: "It's not that we're fancy people, but it just seems that she goes out of her way to do things that just set a bad example for my two boys. There's no talking to her about anything. She'll just laugh it off, with a 'That's just the way I am' response."

> Rebecca, a 41-year-old successful businesswoman and mother of a boisterous family of teenagers, has been uncomfortable in her relationship with her father since his marriage 3 years ago to a much younger professional woman. Although Rebecca admits that her father is loving toward her and her family, she cannot help but feel that he secretly compares her with his new wife.

Finally, some adult children feel that their parents are happy and are pleased with the choices that seem to have brought about such happiness. These adult children fashion relationships with their parents' spouses that revolve around an understanding that they both love the same person.

Not Being Accepted by the Stepparent

Other adult children feel hurt at not being accepted by their new stepparent, perhaps none so poignantly as Samantha, who at age 23 would like to hear from her stepfather, a man with grown children of his own, "I want you to be a part of my family."

> Samantha was living on her own when her mother married a man with grown children of his own. Samantha's father had died when she was very young, and she had always wished for a family of her own. When her mother had announced her plans to marry, Samantha had felt a rush of excitement, and when she was told that he had three grown children, two of whom had families of their own, Samantha began to expect that she would finally be part of a family of her very own. Yet, from the wedding on, Samantha was treated distantly; when she asked her stepfather what she should call him, he replied, "Well, Bob, of course." At the reception, Samantha was seated with family from her mother's "side," and her new stepsiblings sat with family from their father's "side." The next 2 years mirrored the alienated feeling that Samantha began to feel at the wedding. "Whenever I'd visit, Bob would excuse himself to give mother and I 'time.'"

At first, Samantha reasoned that her stepfather was trying not to move too fast with her. However, after a short time, it became obvious that he was not making any attempt to include her as a part of a new extended family. Samantha's sense of loss was keen; she had lost her father as a child, and she now seemed to be losing the opportunity for a family as an adult.

To attempt to deepen her relationship with her stepfather, Samantha must be more proactive. She could invite him and her mother out to a movie or to her house for dinner. When her stepfather leaves to give her and her mother "time," she could ask him to stay. In short, when nothing has changed without action, it is time to do things differently. If nothing changes after several attempts, Samantha could bring up the issue directly with her stepfather and mother. Again, as in the earlier example with Jill, Samantha might tell her mother and stepfather what she herself has been waiting to hear: "I want you both to be a part of my family." It is amazing that so many adult children wait to hear from parents what they can say so much more directly and easily themselves. Both Jill and Samantha were feeling very much alone and waiting for a parent to heal the split they felt; however, such rifts are more effectively expressed by the person who is feeling disconnected. Thus, adult children, rather than waiting for a parent or a parent's spouse to "say the thing you've always wanted to hear," should leave the child position and, as a grown adult, make their desires clear.

Others have been hurt by their stepparents' insensitivity:

Sal's father's new wife, pleased with her substantial weight loss, was eager to offer Sal advice about his own weight. What was initially a simple sharing of a common plight became a source of hurt and resentment between the two. Sal felt that his stepmother should realize that physical appearance is not everything.

Heather was hurt by her stepmother's noting the difference in social-financial levels between herself and Heather's family. Both teachers, Heather and her husband had opted for a life as a teaching couple at a small rural private school. Although their salaries were not high, they were happy with the academic community and their supplied housing. Heather would like an acknowledgment from her stepmother that wealth does not go hand in hand with happiness.

Some adult children would like their stepparents to accept the other parent's family.

Barbara had remained close with her mother's family since her mother's death when Barbara was a young teenager and would like her father's new wife to accept Barbara's mother's family as an extension of Barbara herself rather than as her father's former inlaws.

★ Think about what role you want your new stepparent to play in your life. Then think about what role he or she may want to play in your life. Discuss these thoughts with your stepparent.

★ If you cannot or are not willing to speak or write to your stepparent directly, at least get out your own feelings. Make an appointment with a professional, and provide yourself with a safe and confidential place to air your feelings. Write down your feelings in a journal, and save them, or write on scraps of paper that you throw away.

★ What keeps you from communicating your feelings? If they are so negative that you would never write them down, why are you continuing to carry them around with you?

★ Think about what you have always wanted to hear from your parent and stepparent and have never heard.

★ Write what it is you would like to hear your parent say with regard to your relationship and how his or her new spouse fits in. Write it in a journal, embroider it on a sampler, or just say it to someone else that you care about.

Similar-Age Stepparents: Friend or Parent?

When your parent's spouse is close to your own age, the nature of your relationship with him or her can be ambiguous. It may seem inappropriate to both you and your parent's new spouse for him or her to assume the role of your parent. Friendship may seem a more suitable relationship for the two of you; however, this move toward friendship will not work for a number of compelling psychological reasons.

Subtle role changes in your relationship with your parent would be introduced. The most compelling reason for not relating to your parent's spouse as a peer is that, by extension, you will also begin to view your parent exclusively as a peer rather than as a parent.

You may become involved in your parent's intimate relationship with his or her spouse. Although you may be an open-minded person, the intimacy between your friend and your parent may become increasingly uncomfortable for you. For example, if your new friend should want to share confidences or discuss difficulties in the marriage with you, you may find yourself being put into an inappropriate—and uncomfortable—position: if you sympathize with your friend's disappointments or problems, you may feel disloyal to your parent; if you feel surges of loyalty to your parent, your friend will likely feel as if he or she has been misunderstood. Either way, such a situation puts you in the position of judging your parent's actions, gives you access to intimate details about your parent that may be appropriate and/or confusing for you even as an adult to know, and obscures your original child-parent relationship.

A power differential in your friendship would develop.   Friendships that promote the psychological healthiness of each party have an equal balance of power, with one person not having more power in the relationship than the other. In fact, friendships in which this balance of power begins to shift often deteriorate. In your friendship with your stepparent, there will be an imbalance of power, whether you recognize it or not. Although the two of you may be peers chronologically, you are not peers in the hierarchy of the family, and that is the source of potential conflict. If you place yourself on the same emotional level as your parent's spouse, you may have the uncomfortable feeling that you are competing with another sibling. If you think of yourself as an age mate and therefore an equal of your parent's spouse, then the next step is to at some level imagine yourself as your parent's spouse! Although this desire to be a parent's spouse is understandable on some psychological level, such feelings are dangerous and uncomfortable when played out.

You had not chosen this person as a friend.   When you become friends with another person, it is generally because the two of you meet, recognize some connection between you, and build a relationship based on your common interests. However, with your parent's spouse, the last two steps are skipped. Even if you have interests in common, you did not set out to seek his or her friendship; instead, you formed that friendship as the best alternative to what seemed an inappropriate relationship—that of parent and child.

Your parent's spouse had been your friend originally.   If your friendship with your stepparent predated his or her spousal relationship with your parent, you may have an additional dilemma to confront. At some level, there may be a nagging sense of a boundary stepped over. However, the best way of quieting this discomfort is to shift your position away from friendship.

Spend more time with your parent and his or her spouse and less time with your friend alone so that you can begin to adjust to your friend in his or her new role and to become more familiar with their relationship with each other. Increasing time spent with the new couple will result in either a growing comfort with the relationship, in which case you will feel more forgiving about any perceived overstepping of boundaries, or an intensification of your discomfort, in which case you will feel a dissipation of your former friendship.

An appropriate relationship between similar-age stepparents and stepchildren is necessary. When trying to determine the appropriate relationship for you and your similar-age stepparent, you do not need to search far; the appropriate relationship is staring you right in the face, although you may not want to recognize it: your parent's spouse is your stepparent. This can mean as much or as little as any relationship between a stepchild and a stepparent, but it will include at the bare minimum a polite tolerance of each other and at best a loving parenting relationship that will enrich your life in ways that you would never have imagined possible.

★ Add 25 emotional years to your parent's spouse.

★ Do not split your relationship with your parent and his or her spouse. Seeing your parent and the spouse separately allows you to continue to view them as you did before their involvement with each other—as your parent and your friend —and will prevent you from accepting them as the couple they have become.

★ Respect your parent's spouse's role and title as husband or wife.

★ Think about your parent's spouse in her or his legal role as your stepmother or stepfather.

Stepparents Worry About Adjusting Too!

Sometimes when you are caught up in your difficulties adjusting to your parent's new spouse, it is hard to see that this new spouse may be having the same difficulties! He or she too suddenly find himself or herself as the member of a whole new family and may be uncertain about how to interact with you and your children. Misunderstandings can easily occur between people who are suddenly thrust together in intimate circumstances, even when all concerned are trying their hardest to make the new relationship work. The key to avoiding misunderstandings, and subsequent feelings of hurt and anger, is communication, even when this seems difficult. The importance of conveying your true feelings is demonstrated in the following example:

> Michelle, the mother of two small boys and an infant girl, was deeply hurt when her father and his new wife gave her children three gift certificates from a local department store as their Christmas presents. She described what happened next. "What made it even worse was that my father and his wife stopped by our house on the way to her daughter's, and I could just see the back of my father's car filled with gifts. I was so hurt for my kids. The boys are too little to understand gift certificates, and when she handed them those envelopes, I could see their faces fall. Of course, I had them thank her and all, but it was disappointing."
>
> Michelle and her stepmother did discuss that Christmas about 6 months later after Michelle and her children continued to receive the same gift certificates for any and every occasion. "I just couldn't stand it any more. It was my birthday, and she came over and opened her pocketbook and took out an envelope. I just blurted out, 'Why do you always give us gift certificates?' Her answer simply floored me; she replied, 'Because I was afraid of buying the wrong thing and starting off on the wrong foot. When you seemed to like it, I just thought it was our thing and kept doing it.'"
>
> For Michelle and her stepmother, this talk early in their relationship was very important. Now, 4 years later, they and the children have a close relationship that is based on good, solid communication.

★ If you feel that your children are excluded by your parent's new spouse, try discussing this directly with the spouse.

Your New Adult Stepsiblings

New spouses rarely come alone; they often have children, brothers and sisters, aunts and uncles, and perhaps even elderly parents of their own, as well as friends and other associates. The degree to which you can accept your parent's spouse's "people" into your life will vary according to the individuals and circumstances involved. However, as a general rule, it is helpful to remember that you can never have too many people in your life who care about you and those you love. Also, remind yourself that your parent's spouse and his or her family are now your stepfamily, and, as such, you did not choose them any more than you chose your other relatives. As with your original siblings and other relatives, at times you may be emotionally close, and at other times you may be more estranged; however, deep inside you always remember that they are your family.

A Successful Relationship With Your Stepsiblings Requires Effort

Like any other relationship, relations with stepsiblings evolve primarily to the extent that you put energy and effort into them. Compare the attitudes of Carl and Anne: Carl states unequivocally,

> I don't think I could ever have any relationship with these people. They're just so different from me and my family in every way.

whereas Anne states,

> My stepsister is such a different personality that we would not normally be friends, but she's a generous caring person, and I admire that in someone very much and have come to really enjoy having her in my life.

Emily, a 30-year-old mother of three, recognized that a certain amount of compromise was needed in forging a relationship with her new stepfamily:

> In certain ways, because we are all adults, I would call the relationship we have together as tightly knit as that of my biological siblings. We get along when necessary, although we sometimes disagree on certain topics. I look at them and see some issues that need to be dealt with, and we try to deal with them as they come up.

Stepfamilies spread over wide geographic areas can require extra effort to successfully build a relationship, as Beverly noted:

> I think that we all consider ourselves a family, but we all live thousands of miles apart, and I don't really see us having more than a little contact because of these long distances.

Sometimes adult children need to conquer their personal fears about the new stepfamily in trying to assimilate them into their lives:

> Joan, a 45-year-old professional, was quite nervous before her father's wedding about her new stepfamily. However, after getting to know her new stepmother and her family, Joan found that most of her new step-family members were nice, and she found herself liking them and hoping to get to know them better.

You should expect that it will take time to develop a relationship with your new relatives, especially between yourself and your adult step-siblings. You may never reach the level of emotional closeness with them that you have with your original siblings:

> Betty, a mother of two teenagers, invited her stepfather's married daughter to her son's bar mitzvah. Although the daughter lived in another state, she accepted and attended the ceremony. Betty described her relationship with her as "cordial but not very close. She is definitely considered part of my extended family; however, I must admit that I don't feel as close to her as I do to my sister."

Advantages to Having New Stepsiblings

For some adult children, their parents' marriages may open up doors that the children had accepted would be shut forever. Ellen, for example, the only child of a widowed father, had given up on ever having the big family she had longed for. Now married and with two children of her own, she looks upon her stepmother's children as her brothers and calls them "the fun kids." Similarly, Diana, another only child, welcomed her stepmother's son and daughter into her life with open arms. As she put it, "Who would have thought I'd get a brother and sister when I was already a grand-mother?"

Human relationships come in all manners and permutations. In some situations, you may feel alone, as though no one has ever experienced such an "oddity." No matter how nontraditional your situation seems, realize that others also are facing unusual conflicts. For example, Manda was "extraordinarily close" with her stepfather's family. She had been engaged to one of her stepfather's sons before her mother and he began dating. Manda had to work hard to put aside some conflicting feelings about the man to whom she had been engaged, who has become part of her "family." However, she found it difficult, embarrassing, and uncomfortable to be part of her ex-fiancé's "family."

★ Think honestly about what role you want your new stepfamily to play in your life.

★ Are there differences between the amount of involvement in one another's lives that you all expect?

★ Assume more control over these new relationships. Rather than waiting and reacting, try initiating.

Your Parent's New Baby— and Your New Sibling

A parent's marriage to a spouse of child-bearing age can often result in their beginning a new family of their own. The prospect of your parent becoming the parent of a new baby can be challenging to accept.

Parent's Sexuality

One difficulty is that a new baby forces the issue of your parent's sexuality to the forefront: babies imply having sexual relations, and your parent's baby means that your parent is sexually active. For most children of any age, having to contemplate their parent's sexuality can unleash some uncomfortable thoughts, even if intellectually they understand and accept this aspect of their parent's identity.

Sibling Rivalry

A second challenging issue is your own feelings toward the new baby. You may react with a little or a great amount of jealousy toward your new sister or brother, because that baby, even if he or she is decades younger than you are, is your sibling, and sibling rivalry knows no age restrictions. Donna realized these feelings in herself:

> It's hard to describe my emotions about my father's new little girl. Well, I guess even saying it like that is a dead giveaway. I was the only girl in a family of three boys, and I was always Daddy's girl. I mean I know I grew out of this. I'm a grown woman now, with a career of my own and a good solid relationship with my father, but this baby seemed to throw a monkey wrench into my life. The funny thing is that I know I'm jealous and I know it's ridiculous. She really is a precious little thing, and yet I can't stop the feeling. It's just awful!

What Donna is trying to express is the perceived direct threat the new baby poses to her own identity with regard to her father. The advent of this new little girl forced Donna to look at herself in a different way. Although she said that she no longer thinks about herself as "Daddy's little girl," chances are that she does in fact still think about herself in this way, and her father's new daughter has unseated her from the role she had held for a lifetime. The jealousy in this case involves the loss of status or position in the family.

Carrie experienced similar feelings:

> Carrie was 27 years old and in her last year of law school when her stepmother called to "announce the news." Carrie had always shared a close and loving relationship with her father. She had prided herself on having parents who had been sensible enough to continue co-parenting her even after they had divorced. However, on hearing her father's news, she was struck by the intensity of the emotional wallop she felt.
>
> "I guess I shouldn't have been surprised. She [her father's new wife] was fairly young, and this was her first marriage, but the news just stunned me. I had trouble that whole year concentrating on classes. When the baby was born, I was studying for the bar examination. It just seemed like such a crazy contrast—my father cradling one daughter (of course it had to be a girl) in his arms, while I, the other daughter, was cramming like crazy to become an attorney. My father thought this was

just great and loved to introduce us, but I felt, I guess, more than a little jealous. He had had the experience of having a baby daughter already, and now it seemed that he was diluting the experience of having an adult daughter by doing this baby stuff all over again. I tried my best not to show my feelings, and I do have genuine feelings for my little half sister, but it is strange. I have friends who are already having babies!"

Adult children's jealousy can also stem from their perceptions of being deprived. The child may feel that his or her new infant sibling is receiving more—materially, emotionally, or both—from his or her parent than he or she did as a young child. Manifest in this type of jealousy are often old hurts about feeling deprived in some manner by a parent; children who felt satisfied with the amount of physical and emotional attention they received growing up are less likely to feel this jealousy. Margaret voiced her distress at how many dresses her new baby sister received:

I can hardly believe how many dresses this new baby has and the fact that my father doesn't say one word about how much is spent on this baby. In fact, he seems to enjoy the whole thing, calling her his "little fashion plate."

It is obvious that the baby's dresses are not the issue here at all. The dresses are a compelling symbol of her father's extravagant attitude toward his new little girl, which stands in marked contrast to the deprivation that Margaret so keenly felt in her own childhood.

Feeling Alienated by Your Parent's New Baby

Whereas children still living at home may find that a baby unites the new family and makes everyone feel more bonded, adult children out on their own, perhaps with a family of their own, may feel doubly alienated from the new baby: first, they may see the infant as marking the end of the old family and the beginning of a new one. Moreover, they may see the new child as taking away time, attention, and love from their own relationship with their parents.

A more complicated situation involves adult children who have been unsuccessful at conceiving a baby of their own being confronted with their parents' newly expected baby:

David found that his father's new wife's pregnancy unleashed a host of demons. "My wife and I had been married for 7 years when my father's wife got pregnant. We had been trying to have a baby for almost 3 years with no success. When they announced their news, I felt like hitting something. There she was, his wife, going on and on about how it 'just happened' and how thrilled they were at the surprise. I know that our problem [in conceiving a child] really doesn't have anything to do with my father's good news, but somehow the whole thing seems wrong. Now my wife shies away from going to their house, and I can't say that I blame her. It's embarrassing to be with a woman in her 40s who is having a baby with other kids in college and not be able to start a family of your own the first time around!"

Adult children may find it easier to express the new hurt they perceive their own children feeling at being pushed into the background than their own hurt but may weave their own hurt into their expression of their children's hurt. Lenore, a 32-year-old mother of twin 5-year-old boys, described her feelings following the birth of her father's new baby girl.

Since my father's wife had their daughter 6 months ago, it's as though my sons don't exist anymore. My father used to be over here every weekend throwing a ball around with the boys, watching them run around. Now, it seems that he's just completely entranced with this new baby. I don't mind for myself, but the boys are confused and hurt. They just don't understand why Pop Pop doesn't visit them anymore.

> ★   Use your experience with your parent and your half sibling
>   as a unique opportunity for personal growth.

Instant Replay:
Watching Your Parent With the New Baby

As an adult observing your parent's interaction with his or her new child, you can learn a great deal about how you were parented. Of course, this child is not yourself, and your parent's circumstances and disposition may have gone through many changes in the years since you were a child. Nevertheless, such an opportunity can be a valuable one, as Penny found out:

> My mother had a little girl with her second husband when I was in my senior year in college. I thought it was just great. She was absolutely adorable, and everyone in the family kept telling me that she looked just like me when I was a baby. I realize now that I began to think about her as a little version of myself early on, and so when I'd watch my mother with her, I'd begin to think that I was getting a fairly good idea of the way my mother had probably treated me when I was that age.
>
> One day when I was home on vacation from school, I learned something about my relationship with my mother from watching her interact with my baby sister. My sister, age 2 at the time, was playing with a music box, while my mother was doing some paperwork she had brought home from the office, and I was studying in my room. I could hear the sound of the music box tinkling away in the other room as I studied. All at once, I heard my mother saying, "Now look what you've done!" I ran to the doorway and watched as my little sister stood holding the broken music box, her eyes large and filled with tears. I felt a red rage go right through me at my mother's treatment of my sister; I scooped up my sister and brought her into my room. My mother went right back to her work; she later thanked me for taking care of the baby who had been "getting on her nerves."
>
> For most of my life, I've been overly sensitive to criticism; that day, watching my mother and my little sister, I could see where it may have begun and finally began to put it to rest.

★ Although your parent is obviously not the same with this new baby as he or she was with you, there are probably enough similarities that you can gain valuable insight into the way in which you were raised, or at the very least use this interaction as a springboard for conversations about your own baby and childhood.

★ Use your observations about your parent's interaction with his or her child to speculate on the way in which you learned about the world and how you came to form some of the views you now hold.

Your Stepparent and Your Children— New Grandparents?

Accepting a Stepparent as Your Children's Grandparent

Grandparenting seems to be an especially sticky issue for some. Obviously, adult children's feelings about their stepparents being their children's grandparents will relate directly to their feelings about their stepparents and parents. If an adult child's relationship with his or her parent and step-parent has historically been distant, then the adult child will most likely keep the child-grandparent relationship in the same vein, as did Stan:

> Stan's father left home when Stan was a small child, divorced his mother, and married again soon after. Now that Stan is 28 years old and the father of an infant girl, he is adamant that his stepmother will not be a grand-mother to his daughter. "She had no interest in my father's child, and so she has no interest in his grandchild either."

Charlene, now age 48, remembers that her stepmother was always a loving grandmother to her two daughters who "spoiled them as a grandma will and disciplined them lovingly."

Whether their parents were divorced or widowed also seems to make a difference in how adult children view potential grandparents for their own children. Those whose parents were widowed seem to be more wel-coming of stepparents as grandparents for their children than adults whose parents were divorced. (It is interesting that the opposite holds true with regard to the child-stepparent relationship; children whose parents were divorced seem to have an easier time accepting stepparents than do children who have lost a parent through death.) This may be so because adults have been able to come to terms with their ability to remember the parent who is deceased, whereas this is more difficult for a developing child who may fear forgetting a parent and therefore be more threatened by the appearance of a new parental figure. An adult child with a deceased parent also may have an easier time accepting a parent's spouse as a grandparent because of the simple absence of any loyalty conflicts between parents and/or between the new spouse and the same-sex parent. In cases in which parents have divorced, an adult child's loyalty to a divorced parent may be particularly intense, as was the case with Joanie, a young mother whose parents had divorced when she was a child. When asked about the role her stepmother would play in her new baby's life, she stated:

> She may be my father's wife, but she is nothing to me. Therefore, there is no way that she is my baby's grandmother. My mother is my baby's grandmother, and that's that.

Other adult children encourage their children to get to know their new grandparent because they do not want to deprive their children of the possibility of the "grandparent experience" that they otherwise would not have. Such was the case with Sandra, who explained,

> My stepfather is the only grandfather my children have ever known because my husband's father is deceased. He plays a very important role in their lives.

Some adult children may refuse to allow stepparents to take on the role of grandparents to their children because they are not biologically related to the children. Such a stance may then become a source of conflict between the adult child and his or her parent, as it did with Laura and her father. As she stated,

> I do not see my father because I do not want my child calling his second wife "Grandma." My feeling is that they have two blood grandparents living. This has been a source of conflict between my father and me and is one of the reasons that I do not see him any longer.

The title of "grandparent" can be viewed as an honorific title that one earns either through being biologically related or through someone bestowing it upon one. Obviously, when an adult child feels strongly that grandparent-grandchild is a biological relationship, it would be difficult for him or her to accept a "stranger" as a grandmother or grandfather for his or her children.

> ★ Try to acknowledge that this "stranger" who is now your parent's spouse does have a unique relationship to your children that needs to be differentiated from other relationships that your children have—basically, that relationship is one of grandchild to grandparent.
>
> ★ If your adverse feelings remain too strong for you to overcome, ask yourself why. Try to uncover the real hurt behind these strong feelings, and then work through those feelings yourself and, hopefully, with your parent.

Children are more accepting of new grandparents. For the record, grandchildren seem to have an easier time adjusting to new grandparents than do their parents. As one teenage grandchild said, "I like the old guy better than my own grandmother sometimes." Emily, age 4 years, confided to her mother that she knew she was a good girl because she had three grandmothers, and her friend only had two. Jamie also counts himself lucky to have had his stepgrandparent:

> Jamie was 10 years old when his mother remarried. His new grandfather was a man in his late 80s who considered Jamie his grandson from the very first day they met. As Jamie stated, "He treated me just like everybody else." Now in his 20s, Jamie reflects, "That's what I wanted back then, just a normal family. Grandpa Hank's treating me like a grandson right off the bat really gave me a terrific feeling about myself."

Sometimes, in your need to follow your own direction—a direction sometimes dictated by past hurts—you may lose sight of what is really best for your children in the short and long run. Take into consideration their ages and feelings and the impact your actions will have before making any decisions.

What to call a stepgrandparent. Taking into consideration the special relationship between your parent and his or her spouse, it would not be strange for your parent to expect your child to call his or her spouse something related to a grandchild-grandparent relationship. Some adult children may feel that their children can never have too many people who love them and, therefore, cannot have too many grandparents. To them, it seems perfectly natural for their children to call this new spouse Grandma or Grandpa. However, if the idea of your child calling your parent's new spouse Grandma or Grandpa really sets your teeth on edge, try adding your parent's spouse's given name to the title (for example, Grandma Martha). In this way, you would be setting this grandparent apart from the other grandparents, which is enough of a distinction for you—and your parent—to feel more relaxed about the situation.

However, keep in mind in this "name game" that it is your children who will, after all, be addressing their new grandparent; consider what title would feel comfortable and natural to them.

★ **Chapter 8** ★

Family Rituals:
When Two Families' Traditions Collide

Questions to Think About as You Read This Chapter

- Which family or holiday rituals are you absolutely unwilling to negotiate on? Is holding on to them more important than being with your parent?
- Where did your traditions begin? Why are they important to you?

While growing up, you and your family members most likely settled into a pattern of family traditions; those traditions may now be altered by your parent's marriage. On the practical side, the logistics of family celebrations that now include larger numbers of people are a challenge; however, the different styles of celebrating present an even greater challenge. Changes in family traditions will most likely need to be negotiated, which will mean that all involved family members will need to compromise on some part of a tradition that is important to them. To do this successfully, you first need to understand that such changes do not reduce the significance and validity of the traditions that must now give way. The acceptance of change, the incorporation of the past into the present, may actually pave the way for self-growth rather than signal what may at first appear to be an irreconcilable loss.

In this chapter, I address three types of rituals that, when disrupted following a parent's marriage, can cause emotional upheaval. If you are experiencing such upheaval in your own life because you perceive that your parent's new situation threatens rituals you hold dear, read the stories of the other adult children that I have included and use them to help you identify what you are feeling. Some suggestions for resolving your emotional turmoil are included at the end of the chapter.

Everyday Rituals

Everyday rituals are important for families, even though they usually concern minor details of life. Rituals serve a comforting function by giving family members a sense of constancy and continuation that allows each member to feel that things will go on just the same, forever and ever. Family rituals are a major feature of a family's identity. The way families do things is a code for their identity; the slightest shift in the pattern can be significant because it symbolizes a challenge to the identity of the family. The usual response to that challenge is defensiveness, which can be manifested as anger, sarcasm, or withdrawal. The emotional reaction can seem completely out of proportion to the seeming significance of the ritual to an outsider. Ellen, in the following example, experienced these emotions when a minor family ritual was disrupted:

> Ellen could hardly believe the anger that flooded over her during a week-end she and her family were spending with her father and his new wife. "It was just a little thing, really. We were all sitting around the kitchen table. I had asked her if I could help her with anything at all, but she turned down my offer in that polite way she has. The kids were having cereal, as they always do, and she brought everything to the table already poured out into bowls. When my youngest asked, 'Where's the juice?' she gave him this tight little smile and said something like, 'Juice is served after your cereal.' I could hardly believe it. It wasn't the idea of serving juice later; it was the way she presented it, as though everyone knew that juice was served after cereal. I have a news flash for her: juice is served before the cereal. Period." Because Ellen herself was emotionally involved in this exchange, she was unable to realize that something more was going on than the serving of squeezed oranges. What was at stake in this frosty exchange was the structure of the family as Ellen knew it. What first might seem like an inconsequential event, such as the or-

ange juice episode, can ignite into a blazing conflagration. Ellen continued with her story:

"Now that I think about it, I remember that my stepmother had the
juice glasses sitting on a tray on the kitchen counter, and at first I couldn't
imagine why she was leaving them there. I think part of what really irked
me was that both she and my father began pouring cereal and chatting
while I sat there becoming more and more steamed. I couldn't believe
my father was just acting like this was perfectly normal. Even as I got up
and went to the counter and grabbed a glass of juice, I realized something
bigger was going on. I was just filled with such anger and sadness. It was
as though she was taking something away from me, and I knew it didn't
make sense. But there it was."

Understanding the importance of rituals could help Ellen and others
with similar feelings to realize that a change in the way things are done
underscores a change in the original family structure. An adult child
might have been comforted in the face of a parent's new marriage by the
expectation of continuity of family rituals; now faced with new patterns
of behavior, feelings of loss and sadness may emerge. One way to resolve
such dilemmas is to recognize that nothing you have already experienced
can be taken away from you. The sense of loss is rooted in the feeling
that something cherished in the past is being lost forever. Moreover, an
adult child should remember that family rituals that he or she cherishes
can and will continue in his or her own home separate from the parent
and new spouse. The child must realize that the new spouse has a different
family history and pattern of rituals and behaviors. Marriage is a union
of two individuals with different families. Ellen and others in her position
have frozen the memory of their original families at the time of dissolution; however, even those families, if time had permitted them to continue, most likely would have changed. The adult child confronting new
ways of doing things should remember that as *all* families grow, they
become richer as they open their arms to include new family members
and new family rituals.

Holidays

Holidays are the storehouse of a family's rituals, the time at which specific
ways of eating, behaving, and relating seem to gather. Furthermore, holidays are the repository of the dreams and wishes of the way we hope things

would be. The dynamics of holidays then are twofold: the first pertains to the way the family actually has done things in the past and the second to the hopes of each individual member. When the patterns of the family coincide with the hopes and dreams of individual members, everyone celebrates a conflict-free, contented holiday occasion. However, some disparity between what the family actually does and what a family member might hope for is more likely. Families have certain ways of celebrating each holiday (or a certain collected expectation for how things "should be"), a pattern that has been established for years. At the same time, individual family members may harbor a wish that their personal dreams about the way things "should be" will at last come true on this particular holiday. Add to this emotionally laden mixing pot the rituals of a parent's new spouse and perhaps the spouse's family and friends, and there may be a recipe headed for disaster. Don was surprised by the intensity that such conflicts around holiday rituals raised within himself:

Don didn't think he had had any problems with his father marrying. After all, he was no longer a child, and his mother had been dead for more than 12 years. In fact, if anyone asked him, he would say he couldn't be more pleased for his father. His father looked happier and younger than he had in years. He was taking an interest in his appearance and had an overall more positive outlook on life. Don's children even remarked, "Grandpa isn't grumpy anymore since Lavinia came into his life." Don concurred with his children's opinion. "When Dad announced that he was thinking about getting married, I was just delighted. This new and improved version of Dad would be around forever now. It's funny, but I never stopped to think that things would change in any other way, until the first Christmas."

Don continued with what happened that Christmas. "We always had a tradition in my family that the entire family would gather together on Christmas Eve, have dinner, and together arrange our presents under the tree. Dad just didn't come that year. I couldn't believe it! 6:00 P.M. came and went; dinner was on the table and still no Dad. At 6:30 P.M., I called and he answered the phone as though nothing was wrong. I couldn't believe how angry I felt, and he just couldn't seem to understand. He and Lavinia were going to go to Christmas Mass at her church, and they'd stop by on Christmas Day. It was hard to believe how angry I was; it took a long while for me to cool down and begin to realize that Dad would have a new way of doing things from now on."

On the other hand, sometimes an adult child wishes that a parent's marriage would change rituals that were put into place precisely because that parent was alone. Some adult children may hope that a parent's marriage may bring them closer to the fantasy holiday of their dreams that never quite came true. This was the case with Wilma and her mother:

Mom had been coming over and spending Christmas with us since she and Dad divorced. At that first Christmas, I had been married for only 5 years and had one little child and another on the way. It was actually helpful when Mom arrived from out of town and helped decorate the tree and the house.

Over the following 8 years, Mom arrived like clockwork, and as a result she was always a major part of our Christmas festivities. But the truth is, we've never been alone as a family for Christmas, not even for one day or evening. My husband is really a dear about all this. Then, when Mom told us she was getting married, we both expected that she would no longer be driving down to spend Christmas with us. Were we wrong! Mom arrived with her new husband and set off decorating my house and tree as she always did. But this year, it really set my teeth on edge, and everything her husband did annoyed me. I realized I was taking it out on him and that I would have to talk to Mom before the holidays rolled around again the next year.

Diane experienced a similar situation:

Diane and her husband had been entertaining his mother, who lived out of town, since her husband died 3 years previously. Diane had always dreamed of being able to prepare a lovely holiday dinner for Passover, with her mother-in-law as an invited guest. However, this never worked out for Diane.

"Because the Passover holidays always occur close to my children's spring holiday from school, Mom simply spends the whole month with us so that she can be here for the entire holiday and have some good times visiting with her grandchildren. She is a marvelous cook and knows how to make all sorts of delicacies that I would just have to buy in a store. My husband, of course, loves her cooking, and the kids just love to have her around. But I must admit that I always feel sort of invaded when she comes for the whole month."

"When she married last summer, I expected that we would spend the holidays together, but I wasn't prepared for the idea that she and her new husband would stay with us for the whole month or that we would all come out and spend the month with her. It's as though the idea of the month together had become something she just didn't want to part with. She is really a wonderful mother-in-law, and I would never do anything to hurt her. But we really need to talk about this somehow!"

A parent's marriage may provide an opportunity for changing the status quo. An adult child who has been spending holidays with the parent may suggest that he or she would like to do something different and special for the new couple. For example, in Wilma's case, it is not clear whether Wilma's mother decorated a tree of her own. If she has not, Wilma might suggest that her mother share her talent for decorating with her husband, and join them later on. Wilma might directly address the issue of her mother's possible disappointment by saying something like, "I know you might be disappointed by what I'm about to say, but I've been thinking very carefully about this. For all those years, you would have been alone on the holidays if you weren't here with us, but now that you're married, I'm wondering about both of us missing out on sharing the tree decorating with our husbands. You're so good at decorating, and I think I've learned a lot from you, so I'd like to give it a try next year."

Diane might suggest that her mother-in-law come and "relax" rather than suggest she come as a "guest," which might be viewed as hurtful. In both of these situations, the women clearly wish for a chance to show off their competence to their parents. However, before any changes are made, adult children in situations similar to those of Wilma and Diane might think about how much their parents have added to these festivities. If changes are made, they should be done on a trial basis, and do not be surprised if decorating a tree or cooking a holiday dinner seems oddly empty without the familiar help!

Birthdays

Birthdays can also call up some surprisingly strong emotions; for many adult children, the celebration of birthdays subsequent to their parents' marriages becomes a complicated event.

Birthdays are the personalized version of family rituals. If family rituals are the identifying feature of a family, the birthday celebration is the way a person is identified within his or her family! The way in which a birthday is or is not remembered may call up a host of unresolved feelings. As with other holidays, a birthday calls to mind both the way things were always done and the way one would like things to be. However, birthdays have a particular twist—under the hoopla of celebrating a person's individuality, they also commemorate the relationship between that person's biological parents. In a very real sense, everyone, no matter how old, is a child on his or her birthday, even if only for a moment.

> Lynne, a 35-year-old professional woman with children of her own, was thrilled when her father, a widower, married years ago. Yet, when it came to Lynne's birthday, the actions of her father's new wife interfered with the way Lynne and her father usually celebrated her birthday. As Lynne explained, "I am not a big fan of birthdays. I never was since my mother died when I was 9 years old. I remember my first birthday after my mother's death, when an aunt brought a cake over to the house; I couldn't even blow the candles out, I was crying so hard. After that, my father and I had sort of an unspoken agreement that my birthday would be celebrated in a quiet way. It's odd, but my father always enjoyed his birthday, and I loved making a fuss for him and still do."
>
> "I suppose it really wasn't my stepmother's fault when she planned a big surprise 30th birthday party for me. When I walked into the restaurant and saw all my friends and family sitting there, I felt a rush of confusing feelings. More than anything else, I felt betrayed by my father. It may sound odd, but all I could think of was that my father thought that now he was married, everything would be all right."
>
> "My stepmother, however, is a very wise woman and really saved the day. We went for a walk around the block to 'clear my head from the surprise' (I was 6 months pregnant at the time), and she asked me what I was really feeling. I told her, and, although I don't remember her exact words, she said something to the effect of not being able to stop people from wanting to celebrate the fact of me being on this earth and that one of those people was my father. As I said, her wisdom really saved the day and changed the way I looked at both my father and my birthday in the years that followed."

Ways to Negotiate Changes to Rituals

First, recognize the simple fact that there is no right way of celebrating. Second, remember that neither your parent nor his or her spouse is a mind reader; you need to share your feelings about holidays and celebrations with them. Try to refrain, however, from dwelling in the past; instead, focus on the present. Speak about how you want things to be rather than how they've always been done.

As mentioned above, everyday, holiday, and birthday rituals are marks of a family's identity. A parent's marriage can be viewed as a tremendous opportunity to discuss the way things have been done, the way you may wish things to be, the considerations of the new person in your parent's life, and how you can all work together to make changes in the way you'd like things to be in the future.

★ Make a list of negotiable and nonnegotiable family and holiday rituals, then discuss them with your parent.

★ Take a more active role in holidays, birthdays, anniversaries, and other celebrations.

★ Chapter 9 ★

My Mother's Pin, My Father's Watch: Who Gets the Family Heirlooms?

Questions to Think About as You Read This Chapter

- Does your parent know how you feel about particular possessions or assets? Why or why not?
- Have you consulted an attorney if you feel you have a legitimate claim that may be violated? Why or why not?
- If you knew now that you would not receive what you would like to receive from your parent, how would this affect your relationship?

The disposition of material representations of the family legacy—such as treasured family possessions and heirlooms—is perhaps one of the thorniest issues for adult children whose parents have married anew. This is the arena in which the parent's need to validate his or her new spouse's place in his or her heart may come into direct conflict with the expectations of the parent's adult children. Whereas the parent may view the bestowing of family possessions on his or her spouse as an acknowledgment of the spouse's new role, the adult children may view the spouse as an interloper and any such bequests as infringements on what they view as their rightful property or the property of their other parent. This can be true with items of high personal value, as in the first of the following examples, or monetary or property legacies, as in the second example:

> Betty's father may not have realized that Betty would be upset by seeing his bride wear Betty's mother's pearl necklace on their wedding day. Throughout the ceremony, all Betty could do was stare at that necklace and think of her deceased mother and how her father had replaced her.

> Joseph, a 30-year-old father of two, noted that he never had any particular problem concerning family possessions with one exception: his Dad and new wife, Wanda, clearing out and spending all of his mother and father's life savings before his mother even knew of Wanda's existence. Joseph's feeling was that "anything after that didn't really amount to much."

Even if family heirlooms are not given to but simply used by the new spouse (for example, a family set of good dishes reserved for special occasions), resentment may be sparked as the adult children struggle with issues of territoriality, the preservation of memories, and a sense of threatened entitlement.

Adult children's vehement responses to reallocation of family possessions may be somewhat justified. Research has shown that adult children of divorced parents or living with a widowed parent simply receive less financially than do adult children from an intact family. This deficiency may be attributed to the simple fact that single parents generally have less disposable income than do married parents. Adult children may quite consciously or unconsciously realize the disparity between what they have and what think they would have had if the parents had stayed together. Therefore, a parent's marriage may not only reenliven this old sense of deprivation but also be viewed as a secondary deprivation and a dashing of the dream of future reparations.

The Keeper of the Family Legacy: Your Parent or the Entire Family?

If you are feeling concern, anger, resentment, jealousy, or any other negative feeling regarding your parent's marriage with respect to possessions, property, or assets, stop and consider the origin of these feelings. What expectations have you always had—either consciously or unconsciously—regarding these belongings? How you deal with the inheritance issue depends on how you view family possessions, property, and assets: 1) Do you see them as being owned by the family? or 2) Do you see them as the fruits of your parents' labor and therefore as belonging to the parent now in possession of them (whether by bequeathal or by divorce settlement)?

Some families view wealth as a collective venture, with members adding to (or subtracting from) one large family pie. If yours is such a family, trust funds may have been set up for future generations, or a family business may require that members continue to work or contribute to its success. If your sense of family possessions, property, and assets is not as clearly outlined, you may need to discuss this with your parent. Does your parent share your view of "all for one and one for all," and, along that line, do you believe that assets, possessions, and so forth that you have accumulated belong to the "family" as well? After you have thought through your own position, consider raising this issue with your parent. If you feel uncomfortable about raising the issue of inheritance, why do you think this is so? Do a little more thinking. Are you uncomfortable because you are no longer sure about your sense of entitlement? Are you uncomfortable because you are not sure of your parent's position on such matters? If you believe that you are entitled to your parent's possessions, property, or assets, where did you get such a belief? If you have certain expectations about specific possessions, were you told by family members that certain belongings would be yours? Once you have answered such questions for yourself, you might want to broach the subject with your parent, with the understanding that your parent is legally entitled to do with his or her possessions what he or she chooses, as you are entitled to do what you wish with what you have acquired.

If your parent has a view that is different from your own, try to uncover the origin of your conviction about family holdings. Once you have identified and expressed the source of your expectations, you will be able to move forward to the next step of attempting to resolve any discrepancy between your and your parent's view.

What Part of the Family Legacy Belongs to You?

An even more personal dilemma is the question of what portion of the family inheritance you have assumed—either consciously or unconsciously—would eventually belong to you but which you now feel might be given to the new spouse. Again, determine the origin of your expectations and how long you have held these convictions. This hidden conflict between what you feel you deserve and what you feel you will be given can be the source of some of your negative feelings toward your parent's new spouse. If your expectations were that certain items would be passed on to you, it does not mean you are greedy or spoiled. For example,

> Allison was the only granddaughter of a woman of considerable means. Allison's grandmother delighted in teaching her little granddaughter how to read the financial pages and the stock and bond quotes. Allison's grandmother would refer to specific stocks and funds and told Allison directly during her childhood that someday she would have to "know how to manage such things." Allison's grandmother had died about 8 months before her father's marriage to a much younger woman, and they had not mentioned to Allison any stocks or bonds or anything concrete for that matter. Allison found herself watching what her new stepmother was wearing, noting new pieces of jewelry and crystal with a growing resentment. She soon realized that she did not bear any direct animosity toward her father's new wife but was struck by her suspicion that it was her inheritance from her grandmother that was funding these purchases.

In other situations, a favorite piece of jewelry, a tool set, or some modest trinket or keepsake might have been promised directly by the owner to the adult child. In such cases, the parent must be informed of the owner's intention. Assuming that a parent "knows" about an adult child's expectations is not wise; it is far better for an adult child to express legitimate reasons underlying the belief that certain parts of an inheritance belong to him or her.

Legal Considerations

Obviously in affairs of possessions, property, and assets, there will be legal considerations. If you feel that a legitimate legal right of yours is about to be violated, by all means consult an attorney. But first, go through the hard work of determining what the elements of the family inheritance mean to you. Chances are your concerns have less of a legal and more of an emotional basis. Possessions, property, and assets often become symbols for deeper desires. Use this opportunity to look beyond the pin or watch, lot of land, bond, tools, or whatever else it is that you feel may be taken away from you and honestly examine whether it is the object you crave or what that object has come to mean to you. When you have done this hard work, you will be ready to move on to either secure legal advisement or, more likely, come to an understanding that will allow you to speak up for what you want or realize that it is not the material representation but something else that you are afraid of losing. One caution: Remember that issues not resolved within yourself are destined to be acted out in another arena. So if you are upset or concerned about such matters, try to work them out for yourself—either with your parent or with some professional assistance.

If you simply want some questions answered and have reason to believe that your parent would be upset by your asking them, you would do best to seek legal advice regarding your claims as a future inheritor with respect to the insurance monies, pensions, trust accounts, and so forth that you are aware predated your parent's recent marriage. Laws vary from state to state, so be certain to consult an attorney who is knowledgeable on matters in the state where your parent lives as well as laws in your own state.

As in all conflicts, full communication between all parties can help avoid problems from developing as well as ease dilemmas. People often assume that other people view certain matters the same way they do; such assumptions can lead to conflicting views if they are not clearly stated and worked through. Family "understandings" can quickly become family misunderstandings, as Madeline learned:

> I had never thought too much about these things at all. After my father's death, all his insurance money and bank accounts and so forth went to my mother. I knew this was in his will and was the way he wanted things to be. But, I guess I also knew that he expected that if anything were to happen to him, my mother would be fair in splitting up things between my brother and me. At least that was what he said on the few times when we had occasion to talk about such things. I had no reason to think otherwise. Frankly, I don't think until my father actually became ill and died that I really thought about either one of them dying. Nevertheless, he did die, and my mother inherited everything.
>
> Five years later when she spoke to me about a man she had been seeing, I was surprised to find myself immediately thinking about that

money. Now, it seemed that with her talking about getting married she would have other priorities in her life that my father had not considered. To be perfectly frank, I guess that I'm also a little annoyed at my father for not being able to think ahead, but I guess few people do. I really feel that money was left to my mother, my brother, and me by my father, with the understanding that it would be used first by my mother and then later on (if anything was left) by my brother and myself. I don't like this detour. I just have the feeling that now that my mother does not "need" this money to live, she's going to see it as disposable income rather than a legacy left by my father to his family!

★ Think about what a particular keepsake, heirloom, or asset means to you and why.

★ Think about "making a case" for why you should have a right or a claim to a particular keepsake, heirloom, or asset.

★ Take your parent out for a cup of coffee or lunch and explain how much certain items or assets mean to you. Often misunderstandings arise because desires have not been voiced openly.

★ **Chapter 10** ★

Conclusion

Golden Opportunities Hidden in a Parent's Marriage

A parent's marriage is a time of major transitions for you, your parent, your family members, and your parent's new spouse. As you struggle to integrate your parent's new relationship into your life, you will meet yourself; if you are honest and open, you can use this transition time to learn a little more about yourself, explore how you relate to your family and others around you, perhaps redefine the meaning of family for you, and achieve added personal growth from what you learn. All life experiences can be perceived as "grist for the mill," as experiences that can be digested and processed into an opportunity for productive, positive self-growth. A parent's marriage in particular presents you with many golden opportunities.

Opportunity to become reconciled with your parent.   Many adult children are estranged from their parents because of old hurts and long, unresolved difficulties originating around the time of the parents' divorce or a parent's death. An impending or new marriage seems to serve as a sort of last call to adult children and their parents to resolve old hurts, clear up misunderstandings, redirect their relationship, and begin supporting one another. There is almost a desperate quality to this call to action, as though both child and parent perceive that things are again changing and that time is moving quickly for both of them. They may realize that if this opportunity is overlooked, all chances for straightening things out may eventually be lost.

Opportunity to reconcile yourself to your other parent's death.   Many adult children realize that they have never actually reconciled themselves to the reality of their other parent's death. In an attempt to cope with the pain of this loss, they may have thought of their deceased parent almost as though he or she was on an extended business trip or a very long holiday, out of sight but never out of mind, and in this way, never deceased. As long as the remaining parent was unmarried, this unconscious manner of coping functioned. The marriage of a parent presents the challenge of confronting and coping with the loss of the other parent.

Opportunity to make positive changes in your own life.   Once you see your parent taking risks to make his or her life better, you might be encouraged to follow his or her example, as did 39-year-old Joe:

> When Joe's 72-year-old father, a widower who lived with Joe and his family, announced his plans to marry, Joe reacted this way: "When I heard about Dad's idea to get married, I wanted to just put my foot down and tell him that he just wasn't going to go through with it. After all, we all had a life here together. Dad was a part of my family with my wife and kids, and there was just no reason for him to get married as far as I could see."
>
> Joe had always wanted his own home contracting business, and yet he felt that his job as a manager at a large home improvement center was secure. After all, Joe thought, I am a family man, with three kids, a wife, and all sorts of responsibilities. Joe's father's marriage prompted Joe to look at life differently. After a while he began to view his father's marriage as a life lesson. Joe began to toy with the idea that perhaps he could begin to live the life he had always wanted. After all, if his father could go after something he wanted, even when there was no pressing reason to do so, Joe began to feel that he too could take a chance at change and eventually started his own business.

Opportunity to openly communicate feelings.   A marriage is also a time when parents and their children are encouraged to reveal thoughts they normally would have kept silent. Some of the thoughts I encountered in writing this book included the following:

- I wish I had not been so open with my opinions that hurt you.
- I am happy that you are happy.
- I am angry at you for always controlling family relationships and traditions. The way you did this made it hard for me to form bonds with other family members or establish traditions of our own; now you have abandoned all that in favor of a stranger.
- Despite everything, I still love you. I just can't help but wonder why you don't still love me.
- I'm sorry you've always had so many problems. I know it's been hard.
- You need to stand on your own!
- Congratulations to you!

Tolerance of Ambiguity

When all is said and done, the most significant gain that we may garner from a parent's marriage is a greater tolerance of ambiguity. The disruptions, shifts, conflicts, recognized yearnings, and confrontations of losses brought about by a parent's marriage teach one clear lesson: life is about change. The process of confronting the considerable challenges posed by your parent's marriage encourages further development of your ability to understand and cope with change and uncertainty. There can be little growth in life if one wishes everything to stay the same. Perhaps in no other situation is the conflict between wanting to embrace change and self-growth and fearing change and instability drawn so clearly.

In the end, no matter how young or old we are, part of us always remains our parent's child. This part of us yearns to be at one again with our parents, reaching back toward some distant hazy past when relationships were easy and uncomplicated and the promise of all our needs being met immediately, effortlessly, and magically was still possible. Throughout life, a tension has existed between wanting to be free, alone, and independently self-sustaining and wanting to be close, related, and, as mentioned, even merged with another. A parent's marriage motivates us to integrate these competing demands into one person—neither separate and alone nor related and merged but an individual capable of both self-sufficiency and relatedness with others. When a parent marries, we are once again separated from our parent because the way we have come to know and relate to him or her is challenged. Yet, if we recognize this separation, we also have an opportunity to take stock of ourselves and our relationship with our parent and to reconnect with our parent in a new, different way. In both—the separation and the reconnection—we will, if we are open to the possibility, see different truths about ourselves, our parents, our families, and the nature of life itself.

Bibliography

Baldridge L: *The New Manners for the 90's*. New York, Rawson Associates, 1990

Barnett R, Marshall N, Peck J: Adult son-parent relationships and their associations with sons' psychological distress. *Journal of Family Issues* 13:505–525, 1992

Benson M, Arditti J, Reguero J, et al: Intergenerational transmission: attributions in relationships with parents and intimate others. *Journal of Family Issues* 13:450–463, 1992

Coward R, Dwyer J: The association of gender sibling network composition and patterns of parent care by adult children. *Research on Aging* 12:158–181, 1990

Drill R: *Young Adult Children of Divorced Parents: Depression and the Perception of Loss*. New York, Haworth, 1987

Fine M: A social science perspective on stepfamily law: suggestions for legal reform. *Family Relations* 38:53–58, 1989

Gilbert E: *The Complete Wedding Planner*. New York, Warner, 1989

Goldberg J, Mitchell S: *Object Relations in Psychoanalytic Theory*. Cambridge, MA, Harvard University Press, 1983

Gray N: *You and Your Wedding*. New York, Bantam, 1986

Gross P: *Defining Post-Divorce Remarriage Families: A Typology Based on the Subjective Perceptions of Children*. New York, Haworth, 1987

Hartung B, Sweeney K: Why adult children return home. *The Social Science Journal* 28:467–480, 1991

James S, Johnson D: Social interdependence, psychological adjustment, and marital satisfaction in second marriages. *Journal of Social Psychology* 3:287–303, 1987

Jerrels' Will: Surrogate's Court, 63-NYS 2d 499, 1946

Keshet J: *Cognitive Remodeling of the Family: How Remarried People View Stepfamilies.* New York, American Orthopsychiatric Association, 1989

Luckerman N, Dunnan N: *The Amy Vanderbilt Complete Book of Etiquette.* New York, Doubleday, 1995

Martin J: *Miss Manners on Painfully Proper Weddings.* New York, Crown, 1995

Pasely K, Ihinger-Tallman M: Boundary ambiguity in remarriage: does ambiguity differentiate degree of marital adjustment and integration. *Family Relations* 38:46–52, 1989

Pett M, Lang N, Gander A: Late-life divorce: its impact on family rituals. *Journal of Family Issues* 13:526–552, 1992

Post E: *Emily Post's Complete Book of Wedding Etiquette.* New York, HarperCollins, 1991

Sanders G, Trygstad D: Stepgrandparents and grandparents: the view from young adults. *Family Relations* 38:71–75, 1989

Sauer L, Fine A: Parent-child relationships in stepparent families. *Journal of Family Psychology* 1:434–450, 1988

Schwebel A, Fine M, Renner M: A study of perceptions of the stepparent role. *Journal of Family Issues* 12:43–57, 1991

Visher EB, Visher J: *Stepfamilies, Myths and Realities.* Secaucus, NJ, Citadel, 1979

White L: The effect of parental divorce and remarriage on parental support for adult children. *Journal of Family Issues* 13:243–250, 1992

Wright C, Maxwell J: Social support during adjustment to later-life divorce: how adult children help parent. *Journal of Divorce and Remarriage* 15:21–47, 1991

Index

Half siblings, 83–87
  alienated feelings, 85–86
  guidelines for action, 86, 87
  sexuality of parents, 83
  sibling rivalry, 84–85
Heirlooms. *See* Inheritance
Helpless feelings, 26
Holiday celebrations, 95–98
Homosexual marriages, 61

Incompetence to remarry, 65–68
  court judgment as to
      incompetence, 66–67
  definition of mental
      incompetence, 66
  foolishness versus incompetence,
      68
  guidelines for action, 67
  questions to think about, 65
Inheritance, 11–12, 101–106
  attitudes toward family
      possessions, 102–103
  discussions within family,
      103, 105–106
  expectations about distribution,
      103–104
  guidelines for action, 106
  legal considerations, 104–106
  questions to think about, 101
Insecure feelings, 25–27
Invitations to wedding, 55–56, 60

Jealousy, 34–37
  sibling rivalry with new baby,
      84–85

Learning and growth opportunities,
      25, 27, 86–87, 107–110.
  *See also "guidelines for action"
  under specific headings*
Legacies. *See* Inheritance

Living together without marriage,
      62–63
Loyalty toward divorced parents,
      14–15

Mental incompetence.
      See Incompetence to remarry
Mother's relationship with child.
      See Relationship between parent
      and child

Never-married parents, 6

Oedipal conflicts, 32–41
Opportunities for growth and
      learning. *See* Learning and
      growth opportunities

Parent-child relationship.
      See Relationship between parent
      and child
Physical challenges, reasons for
      remarriage, 6

Reasons for remarriage, 4–8
Reconciliations
  fantasies about original parents,
      11
  relationship between parent and
      adult child, 15, 27, 107–108
Relationship between parent and
      child, 32–41, 43–51
  change in relationship after
      remarriage, 46–51, 73–75
  child as caregiver to parent.
      See Caregiving from adult
      child to parent
  constancy and security derived
      from, 26–27
  father-daughter relationship,
      35–37